CYCLE CHARTING *for* Girls

A VALUES-BASED APPROACH TO OBSERVING & UNDERSTANDING (PRE)TEEN MENSTRUAL CYCLES

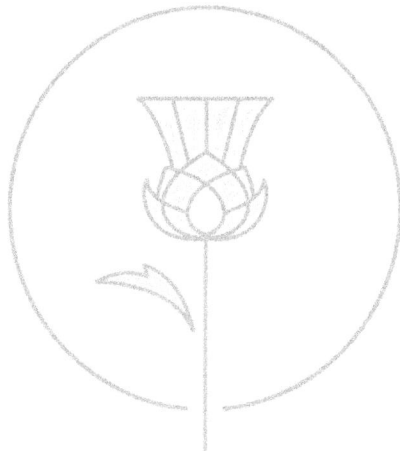

Christina Valenzuela

pearlandthistle.com

Cycle Charting for Girls:
A Values-Based Approach to Observing & Understanding (Pre)Teen Menstrual Cycles
© 2024 Christina Valenzuela

Published by: Pearl and Thistle, LLC
pearlandthistle.com

ISBN: 979-8-9872139-3-3

Disclaimers: The observation techniques detailed in this guide are based on a simplified sympto-thermal approach to cycle charting and only provide information on charting for self-knowledge, observation, and health. These observations are not intended to substitute for professional instruction in a fertility awareness method. The recommendations given in this guide for self-care, supplements, diet, and exercise are not intended to replace qualified medical advice which would be particular to the individual. This guide contains information relating to health. All efforts have been made to ensure the accuracy of the information contained in this course as of the date of publication. The author disclaims responsibility for any adverse effect arising from the use or application of the information contained herein.

Cover and book design by Christina Valenzuela
Pearl and Thistle, LLC

+AMDG+

To S, E, I, and A

> **"**
>
> To be loved is the basic foundation for wellbeing and good health; it's no different for your body.

-Dr. Elisabeth Raith-Paula
What's Going on in My Body?

CONTENTS

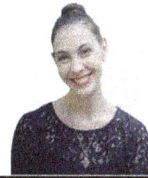

A note from the author:

Dear Parent *(or aunt, grandmother, big sister, mother-figure!)*,

Puberty is a time of new challenges and experiences. This guide is designed to be a tool for you to equip your daughter with knowledge about her cycles—giving her valuable information through building body literacy with cycle charting—while keeping conversation lines open with you about this very personal aspect of her growing body. **It is highly recommended that you work through this guide together** to allow her to ask questions along the way, but of course you should be sensitive to how your daughter may want to approach this topic.

I encourage all parents to give their daughter the option to chart if she wants to—you are presenting an invitation for her to learn about and respect a process which is integral to her health AND experience of growing up! Throughout the guide, though, I remind girls that they are always free to chart or not to chart. Some girls will love it and other girls will not like it at all. Or they will like some parts, but not others. And all of that is okay! As you work through these pages together, it is very helpful for her to hear you say this. Your voice will have more impact than mine.

But you may be wondering: what does it mean for cycle charting to be values-based???
I'm glad you asked!

What this means is that I hold certain values which are reflected through this book and want you to be aware of those values so you can discuss them with your daughter if you'd like to. Cycle charting is simply a way to collect information about cycles and periods, but what we do with that information will be guided by what we believe and understand about our bodies.

So, I want you to know that some of the primary values in this guide are:

- Menstrual cycles are a vital sign for girls' and women's health.
- Preserving or restoring natural body function is better than exclusively focusing on symptom management.
- All girls deserve accurate information about what's going on in their bodies.
- Cycles and periods can certainly be a private thing, but girls should never be ashamed or made to feel embarrassed about the healthy function of their bodies.
- We don't have to love our periods to respect them as a part of our body's design. Periods can be uncomfortable, but they are important for our health and so learning about them is one way we can care for our bodies and our whole selves better.
- I'm a Catholic Christian. I believe in the dignity of the human person, and that our bodies are an important way humans are made to image God. If you aren't religious, another way to say this is that our bodies are an important part of being human. And my *particular* body is an inseparable part of the unique person I was made to be.

I am excited to share this resource with you and hope that it will serve your family well. Welcome to *Cycle Charting for Girls!*

-Christina Valenzuela

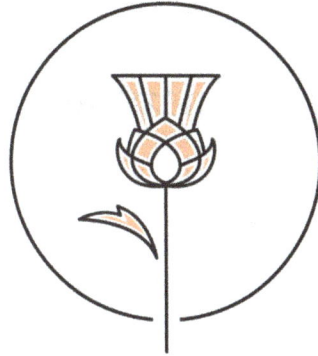

GETTING STARTED
WITH CYCLE CHARTING

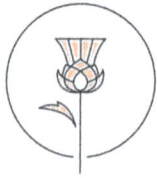

Charting for knowledge:
LEARNING ABOUT YOUR UNIQUE CYCLE

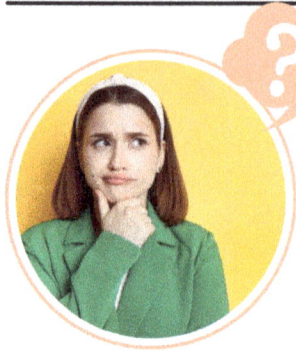

When will my next period come?

Is it possible to bleed too much?

When do I need to talk to the doctor about my cycles?

Is it normal to have different types of discharge in my underwear?

As our bodies go through the process of puberty—changing from kid bodies to looking and functioning more like adult women's bodies—it's very common to have new questions and need to learn new things about self-care.

At times, it may feel sort of uncomfortable to have to "relearn" things about our own bodies. But the good news is: puberty doesn't last forever. And sometimes all we need are the right tools to help us understand what's going on, what to expect, and how we can respond positively. This is especially true when it comes to our periods, which for many girls can seem so confusing and uncomfortable sometimes; but periods are the end result of a really intricate process known as the **menstrual cycle,** during which many hormones fluctuate and can affect all sorts of things like our moods, energy levels, and even dietary needs.

The process of keeping track of body changes throughout our menstrual cycle is called "charting." This is a powerful tool which can give you a lot of self-knowledge— not just about periods, but about many aspects of life which are affected by cyclical hormones.

No girl is ever required to chart...
...but if you choose to do so, you can use a calendar, or you can use one of the special charts provided at the end of this book.

This *Cycle Charting for Girls* handbook will teach you what to look for in cycle charting, how to record it, and what some of the observations on your charts could mean.

Before we get started, it's important to keep the following things in mind:

- It's perfectly okay not to chart—even if you have started charting, you can stop charting at any time! Feel free to pick up charting and put it aside whenever you want to.
- Charting at your age is all about self-knowledge and learning to appreciate your body's amazing work! If charting ever becomes something which causes you to think negatively about your body or your self, it is no longer fulfilling its purpose and it's probably in your best interest to stop charting for a while.
- There are a lot of things we can intentionally control with our bodies, but our menstrual cycle is not one of them. What we *can* control is how we respond to what our body is trying to tell us.
- Don't worry if your charts don't look exactly like the samples! Every chart is unique because every girl is unique.

READY TO GET STARTED?
LET'S GO!

REVIEW OF THE MENSTRUAL CYCLE

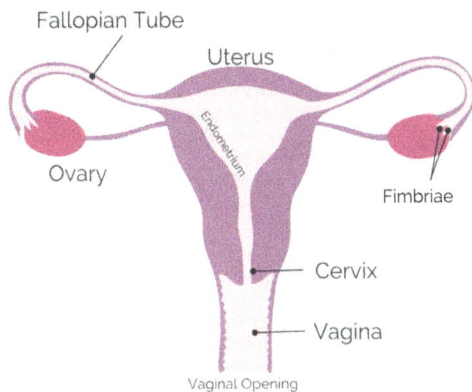

The **uterus** is a small pear-shaped organ which sits in a girl's lower abdomen. On either side are **ovaries,** which contain special cells called **ova,** or **egg cells.** Girls are born with these cells, but they do not start maturing until they are "woken up" by hormones which tell them to begin developing. The story of the menstrual cycle is primarily about how the uterus and ovaries work together to wake up these eggs, help them mature, and release the egg.

Menstruation marks the beginning of a new cycle. During this time, the uterus sheds the lining which had been prepared in the previous cycle. It is also called a "period" or "menses" and the bleed may last on average 3-7 days.

During the **follicular phase,** the ovary is in the process of preparing a follicle to release an egg. The hormone estrogen gradually increases during this phase of the cycle.

Ovulation is the key event in each cycle, when the follicle releases an egg.

After the follicle opens and releases its egg, it becomes a *corpus luteum*, which brings us to the **luteal (LOO-tee-uhl) phase** of the cycle, when progesterone takes over the final preparations in the uterus.

In the Pearl & Thistle CYCLE PREP program, we learn how to tell the story of the menstrual cycle using a story about a Kingdom. About once per month, the Kingdom invites a very special guest (the egg!) to come, and all the hormones work together to prepare a room where that guest might stay.

Hormones in the Kingdom:

- **FSH** (follicle-stimulating hormone) is like the messenger, which invites the eggs to start developing in their follicles within the ovaries. One egg will be selected to make the journey to the uterus (the kingdom).
- **Estrogen** is like the royal steward, which begins preparations to welcome the "guest" who has been invited to come! Estrogen begins building up the endometrium and producing cervical fluid.
- **LH** (luteinizing hormone) is like a herald, which together with FSH summons the chosen egg to leave its follicle and begin its journey to the uterus.
- **Progesterone** is like the Queen, who does the final preparation of the endometrial lining and directs everyone to wait for the special guest to arrive. If the guest hasn't arrived within 10-16 days, she will tell everyone to clean up and start over for the next guest. This shedding of lining is called a period, or *menses.*

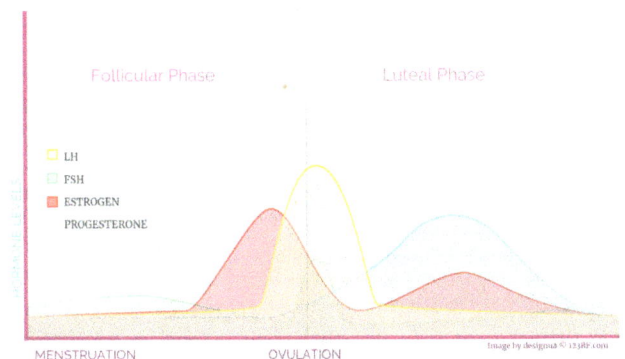

WHY DO WOMEN HAVE A CYCLE?

The menstrual cycle is a unique function of a woman's body. Eventually, it is the thing which will allow a woman to conceive a child and carry a pregnancy. But a woman cannot become pregnant on her own! The process of reproduction requires not only the egg from the mother, but also another type of cell called a sperm cell from the father.

When these two cells join together, a new human life is created! This can be called the "equation of life," which makes it sound very simple but the actual process is very complex. Because everything related to conception and pregnancy is so complex and so important, it requires very specialized processes in the body— not the least of which is a woman's menstrual cycle!

This is partly why we start our cycles when we are young, before we are actually ready to have children.

We technically can get pregnant as soon as our cycles start, but our growing bodies do need time to "rehearse" the complicated processes of lining everything up to create a menstrual cycle. Our brain, pituitary glands, and ovaries need to "learn" how to talk to one another so all the different hormones are released at the right times. This is called the hypothalamus- pituitary- ovarian axis (for short: HPO axis).

It's like putting together a really good sports team: all the different teammates have to do their specific part well, but they also need to learn how to work together! And we know that good coordination and teamwork just takes time and practice.

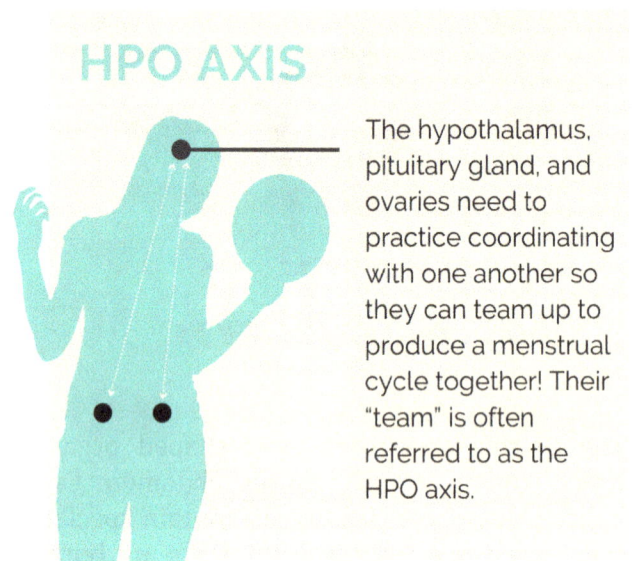

HPO AXIS

The hypothalamus, pituitary gland, and ovaries need to practice coordinating with one another so they can team up to produce a menstrual cycle together! Their "team" is often referred to as the HPO axis.

So rather than focusing on the connection between periods and pregnancy, **we can think about our cycles in the teen years as the thing which will help us get through puberty and grow into women.** Cycles help us create those communication bridges between different parts of our body so our hormones can work together. Cycles create an ebb and flow of different hormones at different times, which carry all sorts of health benefits for growing girls!

The American College of Obstetricians and Gynecologists have said that menstrual cycles are actually a vital sign for our health. This means that in addition to temperature, pulse, blood pressure, and respiratory rate, *menstrual cycles* are key indicators of whether or not our body is in an overall state of health. In other words: charting our cycles can actually help our doctors know if we are healthy! And they can give us important information about what's going on in our bodies.

STARTING YOUR CYCLE:
THE FIRST 2-3 YEARS

MENARCHE (meh-NAR-kee):
the first occurrence of a girl's menstrual period

Girls will start having a menstrual cycle whenever their body is ready to do so!

The average age of starting your cycle is about 11-12 in the United States, although it can be a few of years before or after this time.

Three easy signs to notice which will give you a clue about when your cycle is starting are:
- the presence of breast buds, which begin to develop about 2-3 years prior to menarche;
- the new growth of hair under your arms and in your private areas, which begins around 1-2 years before menarche; and
- cervical fluid, which begins about 6-12 months prior to menarche. We'll learn about that very soon!

You may want to ask your mother, aunts, or older sisters about when they started having their periods: it is not a guarantee that you will be the same, but many times it can give you a helpful idea about when yours might start.

Once you start having a menstrual cycle, it can take, on average, 3-5 years until your periods are "regular," meaning they come at fairly predictable intervals. This is due to the reasons we've already talked about: your body has to learn how to line up lots of different hormones—and it will likely take a few years of practice before your body is an expert at producing your unique cycle.

So you can expect to have a wide range of cycle lengths within the first few years. Anywhere from 21-45 days is considered healthy and normal, but you can also go sometimes as long as 60 days and this is typically okay.

During the first few years, you might also have bleeds which are not true periods. These even happen to adults sometimes! But they are more common as your body is still learning how to produce a full cycle. These are the result of shifting hormones, not ovulation, and when we have this happen, we call it an "anovulatory cycle" which means that an egg has not been released (that is: ovulation has not occurred). We'll learn about these other sorts of hormonal bleeds later on.

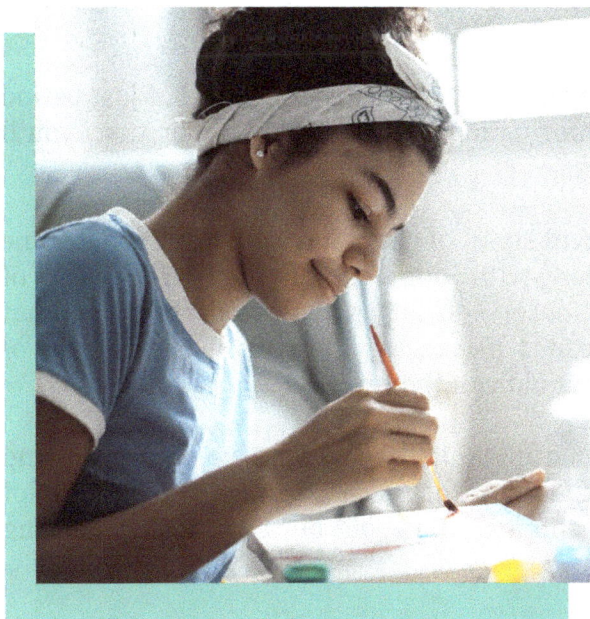

CYCLE CHARTING

Once you have experienced your first period at menarche, you may find that learning how to chart your cycle is a great way to get to know about your changing body as puberty continues. In the first few years, while cycles are still pretty irregular, the purpose of cycle charting is just to learn about your body's unique patterns.

The most basic type of cycle charting you can do is just called **period tracking**. This is the practice of keeping track of your bleeding days, and can simply be done on a calendar either digitally or on paper. If you're using paper (or putting the information in something like a school planner), you can come up with a symbol code to mark bleeding days. A simple dot, circling the date, or adding a special doodle is the easiest way to do this.

But there is a LOT more to your menstrual cycle than just a period bleed! So instead of just period tracking, **cycle tracking** is a way to add in more information than just bleeds. For that, you'll probably need a special type of chart.

In this workbook, we'll learn how to keep a few different styles of chart and we'll learn about some various options for things you might want to track along with your bleeds. In the first few years of charting, we'll simply focus on learning how to observe changes with your body without necessarily trying to interpret what they might mean. I like to say that this is the process of learning how to "read" your body, or **gaining literacy about your body.**

We know that hormones affect many girls and women in similar ways, but I've been educating grown women about their cycles for over a decade and I know that even as adults, we can see a lot of variations with our cycles! So part of growing up and learning about our cycle is just learning about the signs that *my* body communicates to *me*.

KEEPING A WHEEL CHART
ONE OPTION FOR CYCLE TRACKING

First, we 'll learn how to keep a Cycle Wheel Chart. Starting from the innermost ring and moving outward, these spaces are for:

1. Cycle Days *(these are already filled in for you!)*
2. Periods/Bleeding and Cervical Fluid
3. Period Flow and Pain Levels
4. Moods
5. Two Custom Fields, for anything else you want to track with your cycles!

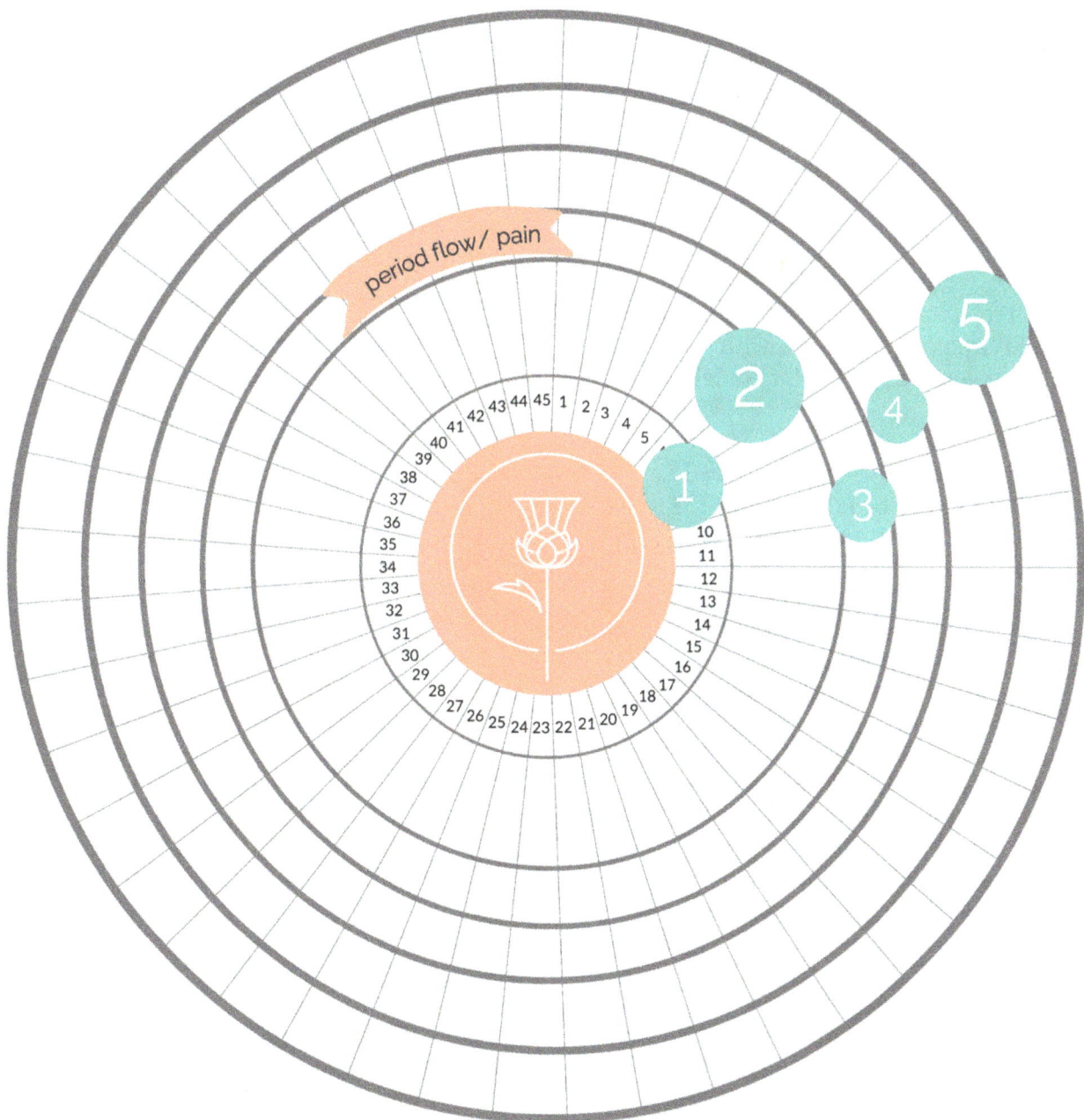

period flow/ pain

HOW TO RECORD PERIODS & BLEEDS

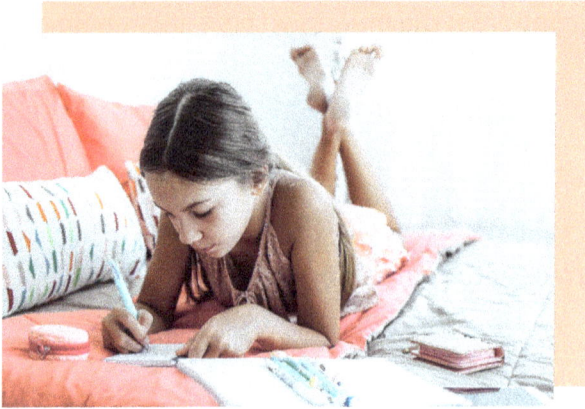

Your period (or menses, or menstruation) will mark the beginning of your new cycle. So "cycle day 1" on your chart will be the day your period starts.

A period starts with a **flow of blood** which can be light, moderate, or heavy. These terms are somewhat relative, meaning that they can have different meanings for different people based on what you observe with your own patterns. If you are looking for guidelines, you could say:

- **Light bleeding** is usually described as being able to go 6+ hours without changing your period product (pad, tampon, etc.).
- **Moderate bleeding** is usually described as needing to change your period products every 4-6 hours during the day.
- **Heavy bleeding** is usually described as needing to change your period products every 2 hours during the day, or needing to get up in the middle of the night.

Spotting is a different sort of bleeding, which means that you may see some blood when you wipe, or see a dappled red effect in your underwear/panty liner. Spotting does not count as flow when we are charting our periods. So if your bleed starts with spotting, it does not yet count as the start of a new cycle.

Noting bleeds on your chart:

Every bleed should be recorded on your chart. When you have a flow of blood, you will color the section red. If you have spotting, you can put red dots in the section on the chart. It is recommended that you also keep track of how heavy your flow was each day, but you don't have to! If you choose to mark flow, use the adjacent blocks next to the red sections. You can write:

- L = light flow
- M = moderate flow
- H = heavy flow

If you choose to chart any discomfort or pain you feel with periods, you can put those numbers in the same box as the L, M, or H. The scale we use is:

- 0 = no pain
- 1 = a little uncomfortable
- 2 = moderate discomfort
- 3 = pain interferes with my day

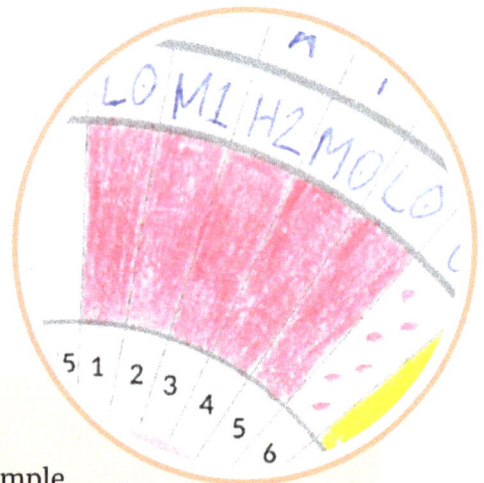

This example
shows light flow with no pain on day 1, moderate flow with a little discomfort on day 2, and heavy flow with moderate discomfort on cycle day 3

CERVICAL FLUID: A HEALTHY SIGN!

As we go throughout our cycle, the hormone estrogen will help our body produce different types of **cervical fluid**. Estrogen is the primary hormone that is working prior to ovulation.

You may have already guessed from the name, but cervical fluid is a type of normal vaginal discharge which is made within the **cervix,** which is the lower part of the uterus. Among its many other functions, cervical fluid helps keep your body free from infection. It is a sign that your body is healthy. But the cervical fluid doesn't just stay up in the cervix: it will make its way out the opening and down into the vagina, where it will eventually come out of the vaginal opening. You may notice a lot of fluid or a little bit of fluid when you go to the bathroom, or as a sensation throughout the day.

Girls may first begin to notice cervical fluid when they start to see a bit of dried, odorless discharge in their underwear. When you see this, it might be a sign that your body's hormones are waking up and getting ready to start cycling! Usually this is a sign that you could start your period within 6-12 months.

You will read more about different types of cervical fluid in the following pages. Cervical fluid is one thing we can observe which tells us about how our body and our hormones are changing throughout the menstrual cycle.

For example, when our body gets close to ovulation, it will produce a type of cervical fluid which looks a lot like a raw egg white: it is clear and has a stretchy, wet, slippery texture. Every girl is different, though, so you may find that your fluid is more watery. Some people also compare it to aloe gel, or simply as a feeling of being "wet."

Just remember: cervical fluid is a good sign of the work your body is doing!

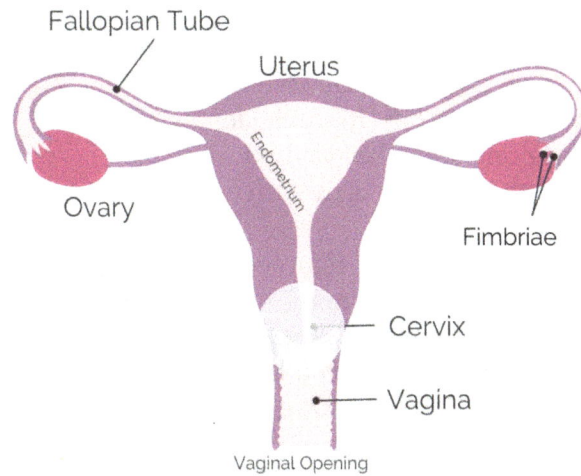

Fallopian Tube
Uterus
Endometrium
Ovary
Fimbriae
Cervix
Vagina
Vaginal Opening

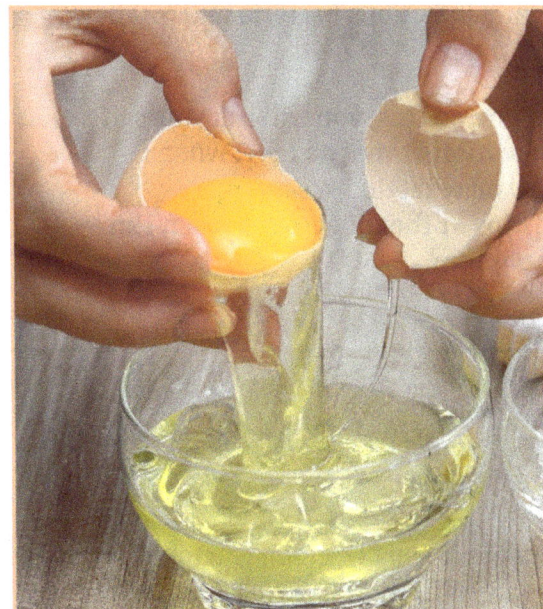

Raw egg white

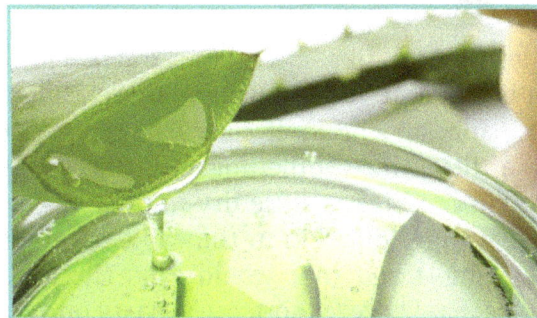

Aloe gel

HOW TO OBSERVE CERVICAL FLUID

FIRST, DO A QUICK WIPE

Before going to the bathroom, you will use your fingertips or toilet paper to gently wipe front-to-back across the surface around the vaginal opening. This area is known as the vulva.

This will help you figure out if any cervical fluid is coming out of the cervix. Sometimes you may also notice fluid come out when you have a bowel movement. This is totally normal!

And remember: cervical fluid is free from any infectious bacteria and totally safe to touch.

When you do this, you will ask yourself two questions: what do I feel when I wipe? And what do I see on my fingertips or the toilet paper when I'm done wiping?

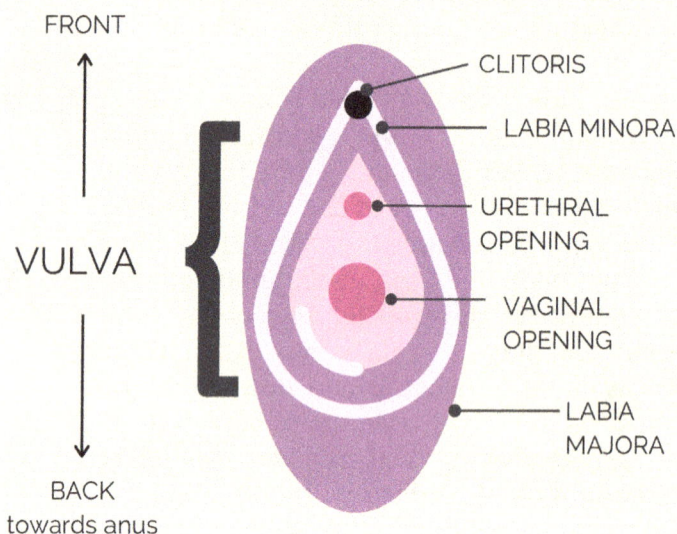

FRONT

VULVA

BACK
towards anus

CLITORIS

LABIA MINORA

URETHRAL OPENING

VAGINAL OPENING

LABIA MAJORA

EXTERNAL FEMALE ANATOMY

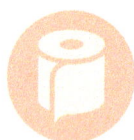

What Do I Feel = What is the sensation when I wipe?

What does it feel like when you take your fingertip or toilet paper over the vaginal opening? We will have **three different key words** for this sensation:

DRY	DAMP	WET
It doesn't feel like anything extra is there. If you are using toilet paper to check, it may drag a little bit. Sometimes your skin may feel a little dry (like if you get dry skin in the winter time!) and that would also be a "dry" sort of sensation.	You feel like there is something there. When you move your finger or toilet paper over the surface, it feels like you may be spreading a smooth substance like hand lotion, or it may feel like there is something tacky or pasty on your skin.	There is something there, and the sensation is very obvious to detect. Your finger or toilet paper will glide easily over the surface and it will feel watery or wet.

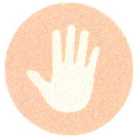

What Do I See = What's on my fingertips or toilet paper?

Then, look at your fingertips or toilet paper. What do you see? You can observe a lot of different things about your cervical fluid:

TEXTURE
- pasty= like toothpaste or a glue stick
- creamy= like smooth hand lotion
- slippery= like aloe, or a raw egg white

COLOR
- yellow
- white
- cloudy (like wax paper)
- clear

STRETCH
If you hold it in your fingers, does it stretch at all?
- tacky= no stretch at all
- slightly stretchy= it stretches, but only a little bit before it breaks apart
- stretchy= stretches easily between fingers or on the toilet paper

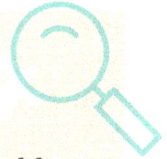

Having trouble figuring out cervical fluid categories? Ask an adult to visit **cervicalmucus.org** and help you find some examples!

GIVE EACH OBSERVATION A COLOR CATEGORY

As our bodies approach ovulation, you will probably notice that the wiping sensation, texture, color, and stretch of your cervical fluid changes! Then after ovulation when progesterone is the primary hormone, your cervical fluid will likely change again.

In order to begin noticing patterns with our cervical fluid, you could just write down every single key word you see every single day. But that's a lot of work! **So instead, we can learn how to categorize different types of fluid so make it easier to chart them.**

Each time you make an observation, you'll want to ask yourself what sort of category the fluid would belong to. In this guide, we have color categories to help make each type easy to identify on your chart. **Each category has particular key words** that will help us figure this out! Here are the key words associated with each category:

	WHAT I FEEL	WHAT I SEE
Gray	Dry	Nothing
Yellow	Damp, moist, sticky, smooth	Yellow, white, cloudy, pasty, creamy, tacky, slightly stretchy
Teal	Wet, slippery, watery	Clear, slippery, stretchy

HOW TO RECORD CERVICAL FLUID

Sometimes, you will have fluid that doesn't fit very neatly into the categories we just learned. You may have something that looks yellow, but is pretty stretchy. "Yellow" is a key word for the YELLOW category, but "stretchy" is a key word for the TEAL category. When this happens, it's ok! You can just choose the category that is *lower* on the chart. So if the options are GRAY or YELLOW, you choose YELLOW. If the options are YELLOW or TEAL, you choose TEAL.

Gather your feeling and sight observations throughout the day. You don't need to check every time you go to the bathroom. At the end of the day, you'll choose how to categorize the whole day... and you'll categorize by the designation that is lowest on the chart, regardless of when that happened throughout the day.

So, if during the day you had three observations that were: YELLOW, TEAL, YELLOW— you'd color that day TEAL because that color is lower on the color chart. If you have four observations which are: YELLOW, GRAY, GRAY, GRAY—you'd color that day YELLOW.

Let's do some practice. Next to each observation, write what category that fluid would be. Then figure out what color category the entire day would be.

Tuesday

6:30 AM- damp, pasty white fluid
12 noon- damp, creamy white fluid
4:00 PM- wet, creamy white fluid
9:00 PM- wet, stretchy clear fluid
What color would this day be?

Color Category:
_____
_____
_____
_____
_____

Help
Lily fill
out her
chart!

Wednesday

7:00 AM- wet, stretchy clear fluid
11:00 AM- wet, no fluid
3:30 PM- wet, no fluid
9:00 PM- wet, stretchy clear fluid
What color would this day be?

Color Category:
_____
_____
_____
_____
_____

Thursday

6:30 AM- damp, creamy white fluid
11:00 AM- moist, no fluid
3:30 PM- dry, no fluid
9:00 PM- dry, no fluid
What color would this day be?

Color Category:
_____
_____
_____
_____
_____

*Check your answers
at the end of this book*

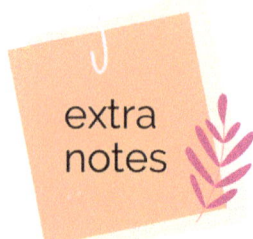

extra notes

1) Looking in your underwear will not tell you about the type of fluid that you are having, because fluid can change consistency when exposed to air. So you have to do the check on the surface of the skin.
2) Using panty liners, scented toilet paper, or period panties will affect your observations. If you need to use a panty liner because you feel wet, that is a TEAL day! If you need to wear period panties because you are on your period, there is no need to check your fluid.

ACTIVITY

Cervical fluid is probably a new concept to you! Try to find some common household items to learn what different types of cervical fluid may look and feel like. Find some materials like hand lotion, aloe vera gel, or even a raw egg white (*be sure to wash your hands!*). You can even mix 2 tsp of all-purpose flour with 1 tsp of water to mix up a "pasty" sort of fluid. **Describe what you feel and see!**

Try to use the key words to figure out what category or type of fluid each of these things might be, keeping in mind that our THIRD category (GRAY) means that you didn't feel or see anything when you wipe.

Yellow — Damp, moist, sticky, smooth sensations; Yellow, white, cloudy, pasty, creamy, tacky, slightly stretchy

Teal — Wet, slippery, watery sensations; Clear, slippery, stretchy

Item	What do I feel?	What do I see?	Category
example: egg white	wet, slippery	clear, stretchy	TEAL

OTHER THINGS TO PUT ON YOUR CHART
OPTIONS FOR CYCLE TRACKING

As you get to know your cycles, you'll notice more changes than just periods and fluid which happen throughout your cycle. Your custom *Cycle Charting for Girls* chart includes places to put information about period pain and moods, as well as two spaces to add custom things you want to track. In the next pages, we'll go over some common things you can choose to chart: just keep in mind that it's all optional!

PERIOD PAIN

We don't know why some women experience more pain and discomfort with their periods than others. We do know, though, that it can be more common for teens to experience stronger period cramps because of the different ratios of hormones as our HPO axis is maturing.

If you experience pain with your periods, it might feel like cramping in your abdominals and/or your lower back as your muscles contract to help shed that rich, uterine lining. If you want to keep track of your body's period pain patterns, our *Cycle Charting for Girls* charts provide a space to do that by using a 0-3 scale (refer to page 8).

Tracking our period pain can help us identify patterns (for example: *do I always have the worst cramps on the first day?*) and be proactive about taking care of our bodies in anticipation of our periods. Discomfort with periods isn't fun, but it's important to try to maintain a positive attitude about your body and your period. Try to appreciate the hard work your body is doing!

Always know, though, that it **is NOT normal to have so much pain that you are missing school or other daily activities.** So if you are having lots of 2 and 3 level pain days, it's worth talking to a doctor to try and figure out why and to see if they have suggestions to help!

Tips to manage period discomfort

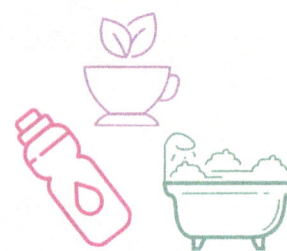

- Drink lots of water
- Talk to your doctor about some herbal teas which may be able to ease your particular symptoms
- Eat anti-inflammatory foods
- Use heating pads to relax muscles on your lower abdomen or back
- Get plenty of rest
- Try stretches and low-intensity exercise
- Talk to your doctor about appropriate vitamins or supplements. There are special vitamins which are designed to help girls and women with periods and cycles!
- Talk with an adult about appropriate dosing for over-the-counter pain meds (naproxen and ibuprofen tend to work the best)
- Take a warm bath
- Manage your mental and physical stress: do activities which help you relax
- For more severe pain, ask your doctor about a wearable TENS unit for gentle electrical stimulation and pain relief

OTHER THINGS TO PUT ON YOUR CHART
OPTIONS FOR CYCLE TRACKING

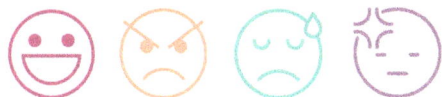

MOODS

Changes in hormones can affect our emotions! Not every girl will experience changes throughout her cycle in the same way, but generally we observe that:

- When estrogen is our primary hormone (before ovulation) we tend to feel more energetic and happier.
- When progesterone is our primary hormone (after ovulation) we tend to feel quieter and more introspective. Energy levels may decrease as our progesterone asks us to rest and take care of ourselves.

At the end of the cycle, our hormones all drop as we reset for the next cycle. This drop may cause some girls to feel sad or like their emotions are stronger than normal. We often call this "pre-menstrual syndrome" or PMS.

Stress is also a mood we can pay attention to: it may be linked to hormones, but sometimes it may actually affect our hormones! If we are very stressed, our body might delay ovulation, or we might have a very short follicular or luteal phase. Paying attention to the effects of stress on our cycle is also a powerful tool.

The important thing to remember is that fluctuations like this are a typical part of cycling! They will not last forever, so if you are feeling bad, it's helpful to keep in mind that your emotions will likely change in a few days when your hormones shift as well. By observing how we feel relative to our cycle phases, we are better equipped to understand our moods and learn how to care for our selves. If you ever feel like your emotions are too affected by hormones, you can talk with your doctor about supplements, diet, or exercise changes which could help balance hormones throughout your cycle.

USING YOUR CUSTOM CHARTING FIELDS

Feel free to add whatever else you might like to include on your charts! You can track hydration, sleep, exercise, or whatever you think would be fun or helpful to add. Use whatever symbols you'd like to keep track of these additional signs. Not sure what to include? Here are a few suggestions for extra items you could track with your chart:

Hydration: have you had enough water today? If you meet your hydration goal, mark it on your chart!

Headaches: some women experience hormonal headaches. If you are someone who gets lots of headaches, charting headaches and cycles can help your doctor figure out if they have hormonal patterns, or if they are likely caused by things other than fluctuating hormones. This is great to know!

Exercise: everyone has different exercise goals to maintain a healthy lifestyle. If you meet your goals for the day, you can mark it on your chart.

Acne: some girls will experience hormonal acne. Our hormones affect inflammation, how much oil our skin produces, and even the activity of skin cells! It is likely that your body will react less strongly to these hormones as you get older. Girls may want to chart acne presentation throughout their cycle to know when are key times that they are prone to breakouts.

Bowel movements: did you know that hormones can affect our bowels? Many women experience fluctuations in their stool throughout their cycle. If you would like to keep track of bowel irregularities, you can also use your chart for that.

PUTTING IT ALL TOGETHER

Here's a sample chart from a 37-day cycle. I've added headaches (marked with a check mark) and acne (a big X) because these are common things that I experience throughout my cycle, but you can use the two outer rings for whatever else you want to track. Or you can just leave those blank! This is YOUR chart, so feel free to customize it however will be helpful for you.

THIS CHART BELONGS TO: *Christina*

CYCLE START DATE: *June 4, 2020* MY CUSTOM FIELDS: *Headache ✓*

CYCLE END DATE: *July 10, 2020* *Acne X*

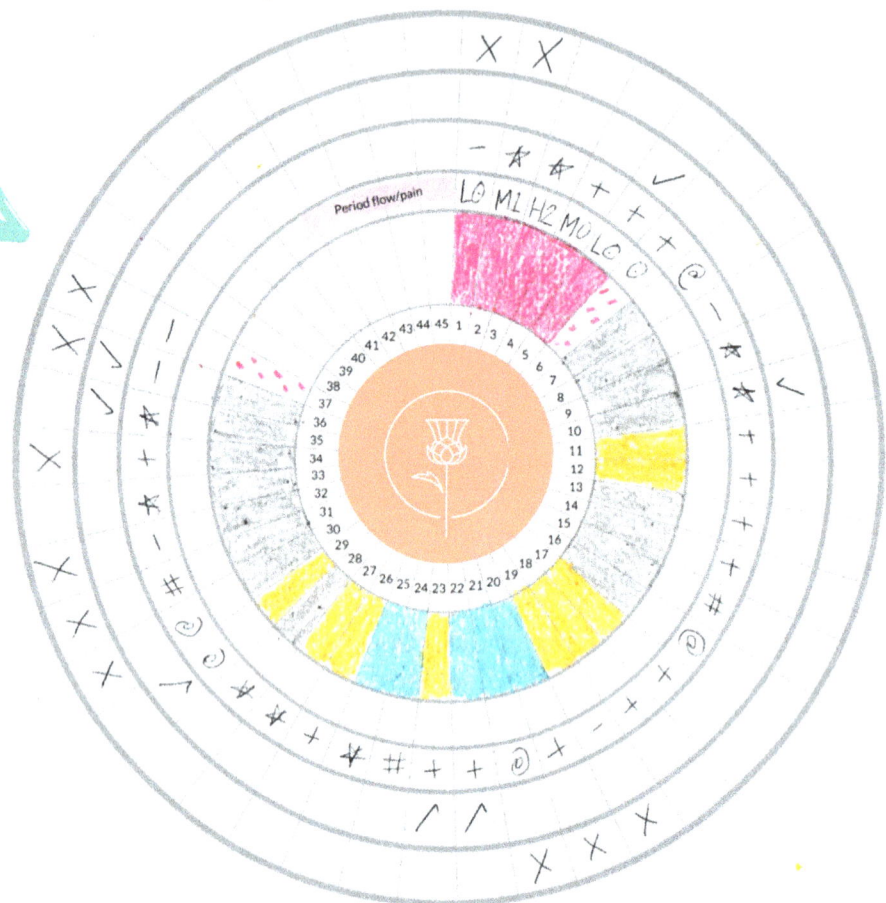

Note that on day 37, I had some spotting. But because we wait to start a new cycle until we see a flow of blood, this day is still part of this cycle and doesn't yet count as a new one. When I establish a flow of blood on the next day, that marks the start of a new chart.

Color Codes:
Red = flow of blood
Red dots= spotting
Gray = dry, no fluid
Yellow = moist/sticky, pasty, creamy, slightly stretchy fluid
Teal = slippery/wet, clear, stretchy, slippery, watery fluid

Period:
L= light flow
M= moderate flow
H = heavy flow
Pain:
0= no pain
1= little bit uncomfortable
2= moderate discomfort
3= pain interferes with my day

Mood:
+ = happy
☆ = neutral
= angry
-- = sad
@ = stressed

add your own!

...OR USING A LINEAR CHART
ANOTHER OPTION FOR CYCLE TRACKING

Sometimes, starting with a wheel chart is a nice way to visualize the fact that our cycles are... well... cyclical!

But some girls prefer to have all the days lined up in a row, which makes it a little easier to record because you're not always going around the circle.

It's completely up to you! So here is how that EXACT same chart would look if you did it as a line. Note that you're seeing it very small here, but your own charting page is turned longways so the actual graph is not this tiny:

June   July

Date	4	5	6	7	8	9	10	11	12	13	14	15	16	17	18	19	20	21	22	23	24	25	26	27	28	29	30	1	2	3	4	5	6	7	8	9	10								
Day of Cycle	1	2	3	4	5	6	7	8	9	10	11	12	13	14	15	16	17	18	19	20	21	22	23	24	25	26	27	28	29	30	31	32	33	34	35	36	37	38	39	40	41	42	43	44	45
Period & Fluid																																													
Fluid Notations	L	M	H	M	L																																								
Period Pain?	0	1	2	0	0	0																																							
My Mood	-	☆	☆	+	+	+	@	-	☆	☆	+	+	+	+	#	@	+	+	-	+	@	+	+	#	☆	+	☆	☆	@	@	#	-	☆	+	☆	-	-								
Headache				✓						✓											✓	✓					✓						✓	✓											
Acne	X	X																	X	X	X						X	X	X			X			X	X	X								

```
                              KEY
Fluid Notations                  Period Pain              Mood
L= Light Flow  M= Moderate Flow  H = Heavy Flow   0 = no pain            + = Happy

Period & Fluid                                    1 = a little uncomfortable   ☆ = Neutral

Red = flow of blood  Dots = spotting  Gray = dry, no fluid   2 = medium amount of discomfort  -- = Sad
Yellow = moist/sticky, pasty, creamy, slightly stretchy fluid   3 = pain interferes with my day   @ = Stressed
Teal = slippery/wet, clear, stretchy, slippery, watery fluid                    # = Angry
```

Note that on this chart, the bleeding intensity is listed with "fluid notations" and the period pain has its own line. Additionally, this chart has easy space to write down the calendar days at the top. It's the same chart with all the same information, just presented differently!

You can use either of these charting formats by printing off the charts found at the back of this workbook, or you could use them to inspire your own custom charting design.

But, there's one more option for charting we have yet to discuss: charting with an app!

USING AN APP FOR CHARTING

There are many apps available which are designed to help you keep track of your cycles. The convenience of having an electronic way to keep charts should not be ignored—technology can be a great help! **However, here are a few things to consider before charting with an app :**

PROS FOR APP CHARTING:
- Easy access to charts at any time.
- No hard copies to lose!
- Extensive "notes" sections.
- Many options for tracking other health or lifestyle information.

CONS FOR APP CHARTING:
- There is no universal standard for noting signs, so categories may not match what you have learned in this guide.
- Algorithms may try to predict periods, or give you too much information about what it "thinks" your cycle should be like. This can be frustrating for girls whose cycles are not yet regular!
- Data privacy or chat features can be a safety concern.
- Many apps claim to be cycle trackers, but only offer options for tracking bleeds. As you already have learned, this is not the same thing! So be aware that not all "cycle tracking" apps do what they say they will do.

As of publication, there is one app which I am comfortable recommending for teen charting with our particular fluid categories and options. **Read Your Body**™ is available for a small, annual paid subscription. This app offers complete customization. It does not do chart interpretations or predictions, and guarantees data privacy. Add the beautiful graphics, and this app is truly a wonderful tool for girls and women of all ages. Here's a sample of the same chart as before, put into the Read Your Body app. The trick with this particular app is that you need to put some effort into customizing your initial settings. But once you've done that, you'll have a chart that perfectly fits your needs!

Visit readyourbody.info to download the app or find out more

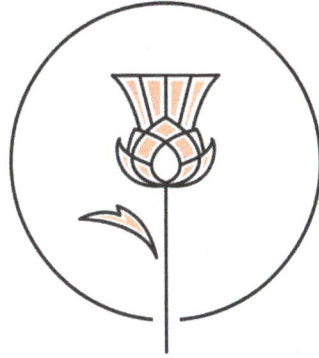

CYCLE HEALTH
FOR TEENS

WHAT IS NORMAL?

Actually, "normal" for a girl who is just starting to cycle is that things are kind of... not normal. **Everything is new for you!** And what is considered "normal" for a girl is not necessarily considered "normal" for adult women.

While grown women typically have a period every 21-35 days, it's not uncommon for girls to fluctuate between 21-45 days within their first few years of getting their first period. This is because your body needs to practice lining up all the different factors which together produce a full cycle. That being said, there are a few key things we can look out for to help us determine when it might be good to talk to an adult.

NORMAL VARIATIONS FOR TEENS

CERVICAL FLUID
Color: yellow, white, cloudy white, clear
Consistency: tacky, sticky, smooth, slippery, wet
Odor: cervical fluid should have no odor

BLEEDING
Amount: 5mL- 80mL over the course of a period*
Length: 3-7 days
Color: bright red, dark red, brown
Consistency: flowing liquid or small jelly-like clots
Frequency: bleeds at least 21 days apart

PERIOD SYMPTOMS
Cramps, bloating, mood swings, low energy, breast tenderness, headaches

*This doesn't always mean optimal function, but this range is considered normal. Not sure how much blood you're losing? A helpful indicator of heavy bleeding is if you are soaking through a pad or tampon more frequently than every couple of hours.

MIGHT WANT TO ASK AN ADULT

CERVICAL FLUID
Color: gray, green, pink, or red (although spotting mixed with fluid can be fine! It's just good to make sure)
Consistency: unusually chunky or thin
Odor: fishy, metallic, yeasty

BLEEDING
Amount: greater than 80mL or frequent spotting
Length: fewer than 3 days, or more than 7
Color: light pink, dark brown/black, gray
Consistency: runny, clots larger than a quarter
Frequency: bleeds more frequently than 21 days

PERIOD SYMPTOMS
Passing out, vomiting, intense cramps, abdominal pain between periods

CHARTING + A HEALTHY YOU

VAGINAL HEALTH

Now that you are an expert at observing cervical fluid and you know what types of discharge are healthy and normal, you are equipped to monitor and take care of your vaginal health. We know that sometimes we can get infections "down there," and that's okay. When that happens, we talk to an adult who can help us with taking care of the issue. But with the right knowledge and skills, YOU will be able to cut down on some common sources of infection and irritation to help maintain a healthier you.

Here are some quick and easy tips on maintaining vaginal health:

- Wear breathable, cotton underwear. This cuts down on moisture which can cause excess bacterial growth.
- Always wipe front to back to avoid spreading bacteria from bowel movements.
- Take regular baths/showers and use gentle, mild soap around the vulva. Avoid anything that is abrasive or has heavy perfumes.
- Eat foods with probiotics to help encourage good bacterial growth, or ask your doctor about specific recommendations for a probiotic supplement.
- Be careful about scented detergents and/or dryer sheets, which can cause irritation and break down your natural skin barriers that help prevent infection.

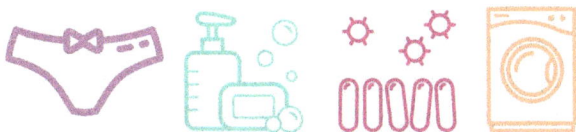

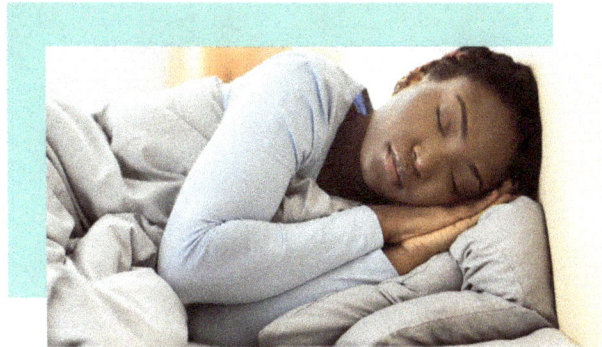

CYCLES AND SLEEP

Yep— sleep, hormones, and cycle health are all related. Puberty is a time when you may feel the need for extra sleep, so don't ignore what your body is telling you. It is doing very complicated and important work!

Keeping a regular sleep schedule will help your body and mind stay healthy: it boosts your immune system, improves your mood, and positively impacts hormone balance. In general, the CDC recommends that you aim for 9-12 hours of sleep each night if you are age 12 or younger, and 8-10 hours if you are 13 or older.

What's the cycle connection?

Many girls and women report that they have a harder time falling asleep and staying asleep in the few days leading up to their periods. At the end of the luteal phase, it is therefore important to focus a little more on good sleep habits. Set yourself up for sleep success by avoiding screens before bedtime and making sure your bedroom is a quiet, relaxing place. During these few days, you may also want to consider going to bed a little bit earlier, which means starting your bedtime routine earlier, too.

CHARTING + A HEALTHY YOU

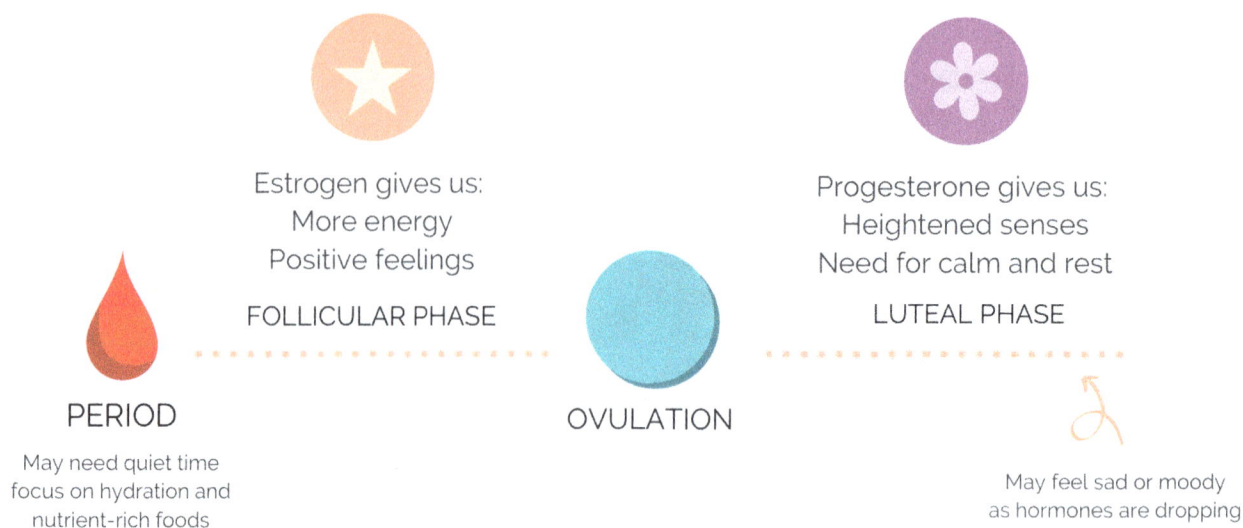

Estrogen gives us:
More energy
Positive feelings

FOLLICULAR PHASE

Progesterone gives us:
Heightened senses
Need for calm and rest

LUTEAL PHASE

PERIOD

May need quiet time
focus on hydration and
nutrient-rich foods

OVULATION

May feel sad or moody
as hormones are dropping

There is no need for you to change your activities and habits to sync with your cycle, but if you want to tap into the natural rhythms of your body's energy levels, there are things you can consider. Any change in diet, exercise, or supplements should be discussed with a doctor who knows you well!

EXERCISE DURING YOUR...

Period: Don't push it! Rest and relax. Stretch, take walks or do some light swimming.

Follicular Phase: Tap into your increasing energy with running, hiking or other things you love to get your heart pumping!

Ovulation: This may be the time when you are most comfortable with high-intensity workouts.

Luteal Phase: Low energy levels may make it more comfortable to focus on strength training or moderate exercise.

Note: maintaining a health body weight with a healthy ratio of fat is VERY important for keeping your cycles on track! Girl's and women's bodies are smart and they will stop cycling if they do not have the right nutrients. To ensure healthy function, take care to feed yourself well.

SPECIAL FOODS DURING YOUR...

Period: Hydration is key for fighting cramps. Foods rich in things like iron and magnesium will help replenish your stores, which are depleted during menses.

Follicular Phase: Protein during this phase will help boost your energy and support higher activity levels.

Ovulation: Estrogen is high, so you might want to focus on anti-inflammatory foods like fresh veggies/fruits and fish to help your body clear excess estrogen after this surge.

Luteal Phase: Pay attention to your food cravings, which may seem more intense during this phase. Your body wants to retain more water, so drink up— and avoid excess salt which can increase water retention and cause discomfort. Complex carbs and nutrient-rich foods may make the luteal phase and period a little easier.

HEALTH CONCERNS RELATED TO CYCLES

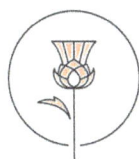

Just like any other part of our body, our reproductive system can sometimes show health concerns. The good news is that by learning how to observe your unique cycles, you will be well-equipped to share valuable information with your doctor if something does come up! We have said before in this guide that you should talk to a trusted adult whenever your cycles show signs that they are outside of normal range. Now, let's talk about some of the issues that teens might face with regards to cycles.

EXERCISE-INDUCED AMENORRHEA

After we've started having periods, it is sometimes possible for those period bleeds to disappear again! When this happens, it is called **amenorrhea**. While it may be nice to not have to worry about periods for a while, we must remember that our cycles are a big indicator of our overall health. That means that if our bleeds stop, it likely indicates a health issue!

The most common form of amenorrhea is caused by our body entering a state of "starvation." If we are not eating enough or are exercising too much, our body will think that we are starving and will do something very smart: it will conserve energy and nutrients by hitting "pause" on our menstrual cycle. After all, a starving woman is not likely to be able to nourish a growing baby anyway!

But this can carry long-term consequences for our bodies and can even make us more prone to injuries like stress fractures in the short-term. Cycles and their accompanying hormones are crucial to helping us grow and develop into adult women. So if your period has stopped entirely, it's important to talk to your doctor and it also might be important to talk with coaches to ensure that you are training optimally for your cycling body.

If you're interested in learning more about the growing community of women athletes who are embracing the cyclical power of their bodies for training and performance, check out fierceathlete.org

PCOS

Polycystic ovary syndrome (PCOS) is a condition which can cause irregular periods and has a number of different symptoms which can vary from girl to girl! Down the road, PCOS can make it difficult to be able to get pregnant and can come with other health complications. Its precise cause is unknown.

Some of the symptoms associated with PCOS are:

- *hirsutism*- hair growth in areas like the face, stomach, chest, or fingers/toes
- heavy or frequent periods
- anovulatory bleeding
- very long cycles, or high variability between cycle lengths
- weight gain
- insulin resistance
- many cysts in the ovaries (which can only be diagnosed with ultrasound)

As with all of these other health issues, it's important to speak with your doctor about investigating if you have these symptoms. There are many other symptoms which we have not listed here, and it's possible that you may have only some of them. This means that PCOS can sometimes be hard to diagnose, especially in the teen years.

But the good news is that you are already learning about keeping a chart! This can be a hugely valuable tool in helping your doctor assess different symptoms and even target treatment towards your unique presentation of PCOS.

HEALTH CONCERNS RELATED TO CYCLES

PMS/PMDD

Premenstrual syndrome (PMS) is kind of a fancy way doctors refer to the common symptoms women experience at the end of our luteal phase and the first fews days of our period. We have already seen that our energy levels, dietary needs, and emotions can be impacted by shifting hormones, so it should be no surprise that many women experience different sorts of food cravings, fatigue, or mood changes as our period approaches. Along with these symptoms we may also feel breast tenderness, bloating, acne, headaches, or a number of other issues. As someone who is equipped to chart her cycles, you can make note of these symptoms and observe when they happen relative to the start of your period and how long they last after your period has started. For many of us, PMS symptoms are fairly manageable with a little bit of intentional rest, nutrition, and self-care.

However, if any of our PMS symptoms reach a point where they begin to interfere with our ability to engage in daily life, it's possible that we may instead have PMDD—**premenstrual dysphoric disorder.**

PMDD includes both physical and mental health components which should both be taken seriously. Treatment will vary based on individual symptoms and severity, so it's important to be very honest with your doctor about any struggles you are having.

The key thing to remember about PMDD is that it is associated with a **temporary** change in our cycle symptoms. So if you have any physical or mental health concerns that begin within 2 weeks of your period and subside after a few days of your period starting, that is a very good indicator that

they are probably related to PMDD.

It can be very frustrating to feel that we lack control over our emotions and our bodies, but just remember that it's not "in your head." The symptoms are very real and so it's important to treat PMDD like any other medical diagnosis: by listening to your body's needs and following the advice of your doctor.

ANEMIA

Anemia is a condition caused when the number of healthy red blood cells is too low. It's fairly common for teens to be anemic because rapid growth spurts make it hard for our bodies to keep up!

Unfortunately, anemia can also be caused by heavy periods or by frequent bleeding episodes, so teenage girls are especially prone to this condition.

Symptoms may include:
- fatigue
- pale or yellowish-colored skin
- light-headedness (feeling dizzy or faint)
- rapid heart rate

Because anemia is also related to iron deficiency, another common symptom may also be the urge to chew ice—a symptom called *pagophagia.*

Be sure to ask your doctor if you have these symptoms. Most times, anemia can be confirmed or ruled out by a simple blood test (which includes checking for both iron AND ferritin) and can be managed with proper diet and nutrients.

HEALTH CONCERNS RELATED TO CYCLES

ENDOMETRIOSIS

This condition occurs when a type of tissue which is very similar to the endometrial lining in your uterus begins to grow outside of the uterine cavity. It can happen anywhere in the body, but it is most common within the abdominal area around your uterus. Endometriosis is often accompanied by painful cramps and irregular bleeding, which could mean heavy bleeding, periods lasting longer than seven days or bleeding/spotting between periods. Because the tissue can grow in different places, some women also report that they have pain with bowel movements or urination.

If left untreated, endometriosis can continue to get worse, causing more discomfort and symptoms. It is also possible for endometriosis to damage parts of the reproductive system and make it difficult for women to have children. There are different stages of endometriosis and many options for management and treatment depending on your particular needs, so be sure to speak with a doctor if you experience any of these symptoms.

VAGINAL INFECTION

Overgrowth of naturally-occurring yeast or bacteria can be a source of infection within the vagina. Girls who are comfortable identifying healthy cervical fluid patterns can fairly easily identify many common vaginal infections simply by noticing a change in vaginal discharge. Always be sure to tell your doctor if you notice changes! You can refer to page 20 of this guide for a review on some specific things to watch out for.

For many women these infections are temporary, but others may notice that they are prone to having specific types on a regular basis. If you find that you are getting frequent infections, be sure to communicate this to your doctor and check page 21 for some ideas about preventive measures you can consider.

Need help finding a doctor who will work with your chart? Try these resources!

My Catholic Doctor: links to RRM for Family Planning, but can be applied to teens mycatholicdoctor.com/our-services/family-planning/

St. Paul VI Institute: National Hormone Lab, the hub for NaProTECHNOLOGY™ in the USA, can provide hormonal screening even with samples collected across state lines. popepaulvi.com/laboratory/

FEMM Medical Provider Directory: you can search by location and specialty. femmhealth.org/medical-providers/

Fertility Science Institute: provides a list of doctors who are trained in charting methods (also known as Fertility Awareness Based Methods) and medical allies, who may not have direct training but are supportive of charting for health! fertilityscienceinstitute.org/directory/

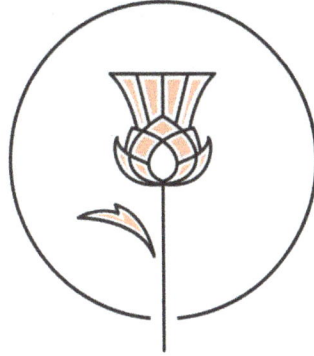

ADVANCED CYCLE CHARTING OPTIONS

CYCLE CHANGES
AFTER THE FIRST FEW YEARS

Once your body has had a lot of practice with cycling, you may notice a few changes: periods might get a little bit lighter and more consistent. Cramps might decrease, and your cycles may become more "regular," meaning they happen at fairly predictable intervals.

As your HPO axis matures and your body gets even better at producing this complicated cycle, it's possible to still notice some variations—but after the first few years, most girls' cycles typically become shorter, occurring closer to every 30 days rather than extending 45+ days. You might experience less pain with cramps, and you may feel like your body has settled into a pattern with your bleeds so you tend to know what to expect. These are all things you can observe externally, but there is another change which you can't observe unless you know how to look for it: **your body may now be ovulating regularly!**

In the first section, we were simply charting to observe patterns of different signs; but this advanced section of the charting guide will teach you specifically how to look for signs of ovulation—which can be a key indicator of your overall health and a great way to learn more about your body.

CHARTING FOR OVULATION

First of all, it is important to remember that you are not required to chart your cycles! Charting is a personal decision which has many benefits, but it can also be a challenge to keep a chart on a regular basis. You should feel free to chart—or not—whenever you feel comfortable. If you decide to chart, you'll see the most benefit by choosing to chart in a way that helps you identify when ovulation is happening within your unique cycle.

Checking for ovulation can tell us all sorts of things like:

- when might my next period start?
- is my body healthy in its ovulation patterns?
- are there any signs of cycle abnormalities that I should talk to the doctor about?
- how well are my hormones lining up and working together?
- do I notice any changes in my moods, energy levels, or body needs that are directly related to the timing of ovulation?

Learning about ovulation and how it relates to our cycle phases can give us a lot of helpful information! So let's add a few new charting skills to our toolkit, shall we?

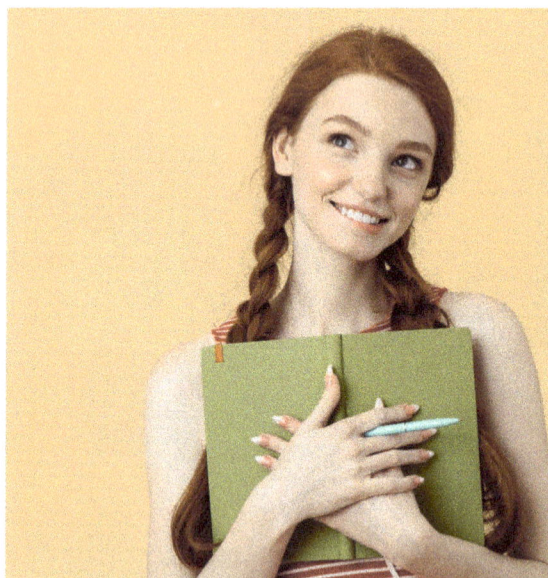

WHY IS OVULATION SO IMPORTANT?

OVULATION & PROGESTERONE

Remember that after ovulation, you enter the **luteal phase** of your cycle. This is when your body produces progesterone. Without ovulation, there's still estrogen (we make a few different types in our bodies!) BUT there's no progesterone. This is important because progesterone plays a key part in boosting our immune system, stimulating growth of bones and muscle, limiting androgens (so-called "male" hormones, even though both girls and boys naturally have them!), and much more. **In short: it's a super hormone with a lot of healthy benefits!**

We've also said that the menstrual cycle, with its symphony of different hormones at different times, is what will eventually allow a woman to carry a pregnancy.

If one of the eggs from ovulation were to meet with a sperm cell (a special type of cell produced by men) and produce a baby, it would take about 10 days for this new human life to travel down the fallopian tube and implant within the uterus. Progesterone wants to give the body enough time to patiently wait for the guest, so it exerts a **negative feedback loop** on some of the other hormones. As long as progesterone is around, FSH cannot send any more invitation messages. Eventually, the *corpus luteum* begins to break down and no longer produces enough progesterone to hold off the other hormones, at which point estrogen and progesterone levels drop and a period starts.

We therefore know that having progesterone around for about 10-16 days is a good indication of a pretty healthy menstrual cycle, because that's a good amount of time to be waiting for implantation to happen. And we also know that having **a fairly consistent luteal phase length** is also a great indication of cycle health, too!

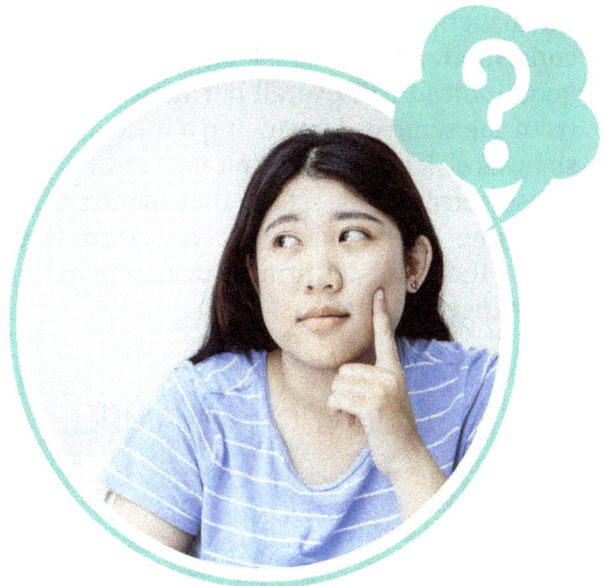

Wait, so if the luteal phase is pretty consistent, why would my cycle length change?

It's all about ovulation: Your body is very smart. Sometimes your body knows that it's not a great time to invite a guest— you're stressed out, you haven't been eating well, you name it. In this case, your body may actually decide to wait a little longer before ovulating. Other times, ovulation is delayed simply because your body is still learning the complicated rhythms of hormone secretion, even after a few years of producing a menstrual cycle. Our body can also ovulate early because illness, stress, or some other factor impacts your body's hormone production.

This is why ovulation is such a powerful sign to be able to observe— it can tell you a lot about what is going on in your body. **But a word of clarification:** all of the things we are about to learn will help us verify that ovulation has already happened— it's very hard to pinpoint the exact day of ovulation. Therefore we can't know exact follicular and luteal phase lengths with current at-home observation techniques.

WHAT WE CAN LEARN
FROM CHARTING CYCLES TO LOOK FOR OVULATION

One benefit of charting for ovulation is that you can check to **see if your luteal phase is relatively consistent.** A predicable length to your luteal phase, even if your cycles are varying in length, is a good indicator of overall hormonal health. Look at the examples below: these represent cycles from the same girl, spanning a little over three months. Maybe in the example of early ovulation, she was sick during the first part of her cycle. Maybe the delayed ovulation was due to some extra stress surrounding school that month. But because she was able to identify ovulation and see a consistent luteal phase, she knows not to worry about the differences in cycle lengths. And she knows that after confirming ovulation has happened, she might have a predictable amount of time before her period starts.

EARLY OVULATION- EXAMPLE

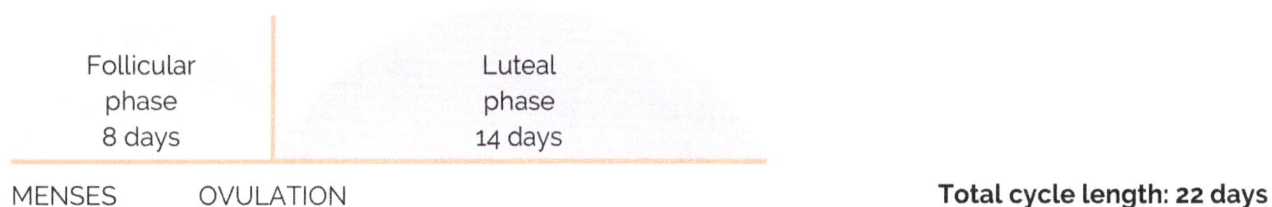

Follicular phase 8 days	Luteal phase 14 days
MENSES OVULATION	**Total cycle length: 22 days**

TYPICAL OVULATION- EXAMPLE

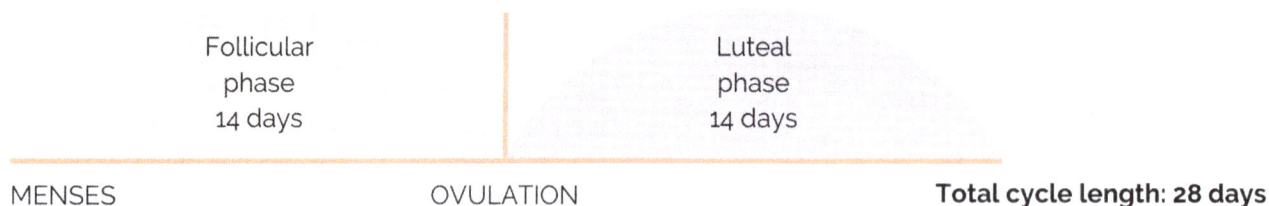

Follicular phase 14 days	Luteal phase 14 days
MENSES OVULATION	**Total cycle length: 28 days**

DELAYED OVULATION- EXAMPLE

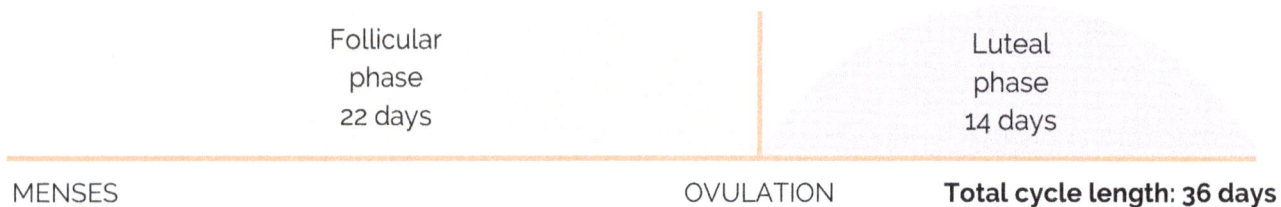

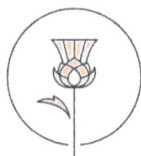

Follicular phase 22 days	Luteal phase 14 days
MENSES OVULATION	**Total cycle length: 36 days**

Again, note that in these examples we have a fictional world in which she can know the exact day she ovulated— a "consistent" luteal phase for you will likely be a small range (e.g., 12-14 days) after we are able to verify that ovulation has passed.

WHAT WE CAN LEARN
FROM CHARTING CYCLES TO LOOK FOR OVULATION

Another thing we can learn from charting for ovulation is that **not all cycles are the same**—even if they are the same length! Look at these examples, all from bleeds that were 28 days apart.

Girl A= 28-day cycle

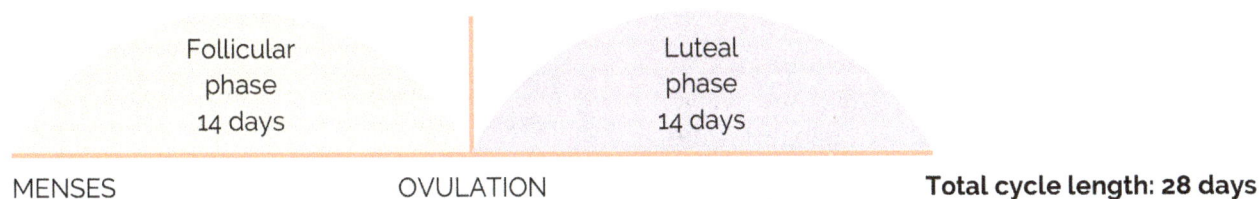

Follicular phase 14 days

Luteal phase 14 days

MENSES — OVULATION — **Total cycle length: 28 days**

Girl B= 28-day cycle

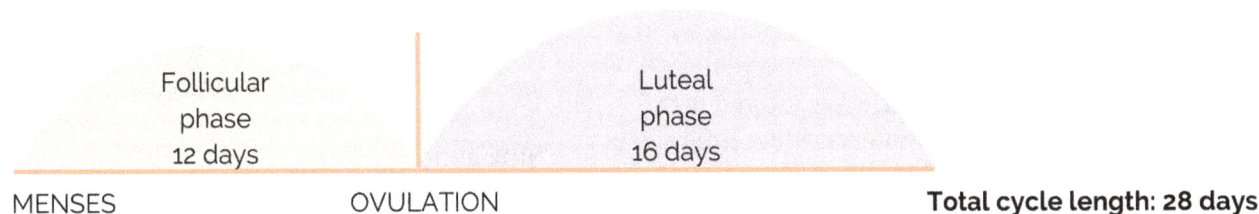

Follicular phase 12 days

Luteal phase 16 days

MENSES — OVULATION — **Total cycle length: 28 days**

Girl C= 28-day cycle

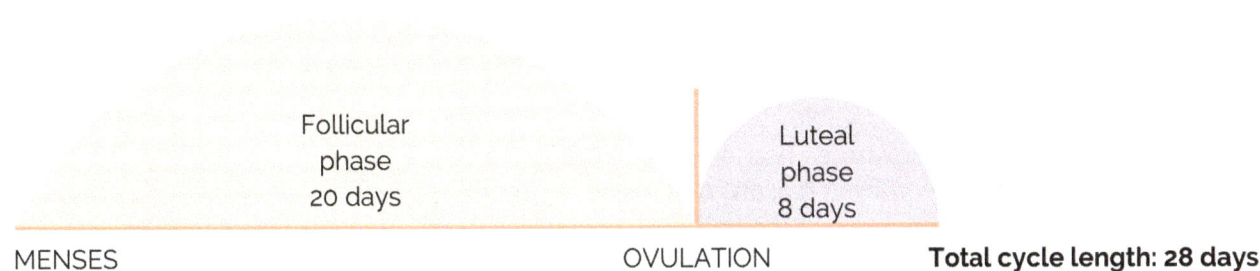

Follicular phase 20 days

Luteal phase 8 days

MENSES — OVULATION — **Total cycle length: 28 days**

Girl D= 28-day cycle?

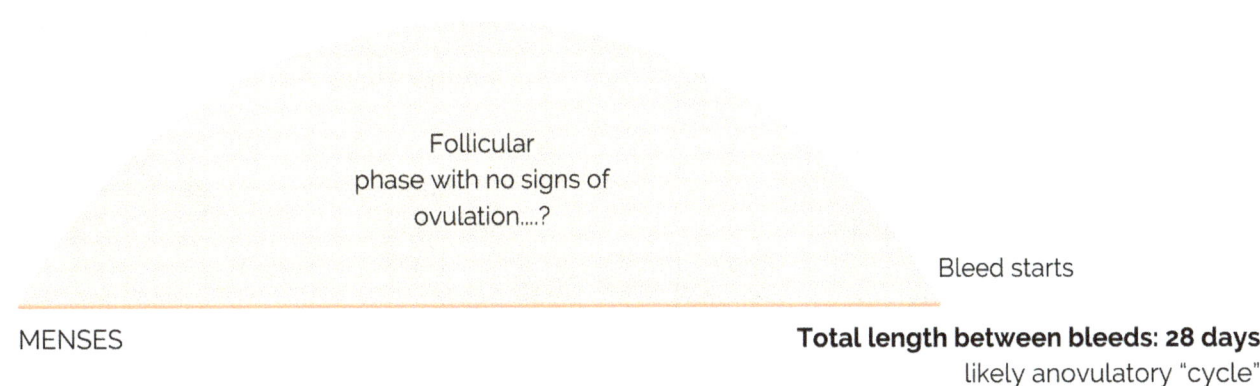

Follicular phase with no signs of ovulation....?

Bleed starts

MENSES — **Total length between bleeds: 28 days**
likely anovulatory "cycle"

ANOVULATORY "CYCLES"

WHAT ARE THEY?

It's a little bit misleading to call something an anovulatory "cycle," because you can't have a menstrual cycle without a period. And you can't have a period without ovulation, because a true period is specifically the type of bleed which is caused by the withdrawal of both progesterone and estrogen. And we've seen that you can't make progesterone without ovulation. So, an "anovulatory cycle" is when your body has a bleed which is not actually a period. So... if it's not caused by the drop in those two hormones, what is it?

Anovulatory bleeds can happen in response to estrogen activity in the follicular phase. Sometimes we'll have a little bit of red or brown color mixed in with our cervical fluid, which is just a normal variation known as "ovulation spotting." Other times, estrogen can be a bit of an over-achiever and stimulate *too much* growth of our endometrial lining in the uterus. In these cases, the body may shed some of that extra lining. This might be called an **estrogen breakthrough bleed**.

Or sometimes, a growing follicle will be producing estrogen in the ovary as it tries to mature the egg. But for whatever reason, the follicle doesn't end up maturing and isn't able to release its egg. Instead, it sort of "fizzles out" and you'll have a drop in estrogen which causes a type of bleed called an **estrogen withdrawal bleed.**

HOW TO CHART:

Unless you've been charting to look for ovulation, it can be hard to know whether a bleed you are experiencing is actually menses. For the most part, we don't worry about anovulatory bleeds within the first 2-3 years of getting your period, because we know it takes time for the HPO axis to mature. And even after that time, anovulatory bleeds can still be fairly normal.

If you are charting for ovulation, you can learn to identify when you might be having these anovulatory bleeds, though! If you experience a bleed which was not preceded by any of the signs of ovulation we are going to learn, you can keep going with the same chart if you have enough room, or you can go to the next chart and just mark them as part A and part B of the same cycle.

WHAT IF I HAVE A LOT OF THEM?

If you are experiencing many bleeds which do not seem to have signs of ovulation, you can check with your doctor to see if there is a reason why you might be having hormonal bleeds which are not true periods.

Think about whether you've had:
- change in diet (especially within the past 3 months)
- change in exercise
- drastic weight loss or gain
- increased stress levels

...or anything else which might impact your body's ability to cycle.

Also pay attention to any increase in headaches, mood changes, cramping, or other physical signs of discomfort which could help your doctor pinpoint the issue.

There are many reasons why a healthy, cycling woman may sometimes experience these anovulatory bleeds! But if they become too common, it is always a good idea to check things out.

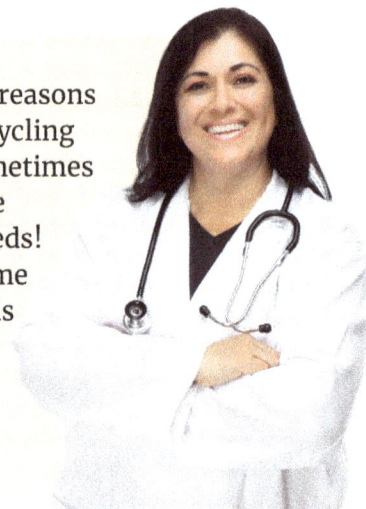

OBSERVING SIGNS OF OVULATION

CERVICAL FLUID: WE'VE LEARNED THIS ALREADY!

Throughout your cycle, estrogen contributes to the production of cervical fluid, which is made in the cervical crypts that line the cervix. This fluid eventually flows out to the vaginal opening. Cervical fluid can be observed externally when you go to the bathroom, or can be felt throughout the day. As you get closer to ovulation, your cervical fluid will change color and consistency because of the increased amount of estrogen. After ovulation, cervical fluid will change again. You have already learned how to chart cervical fluid in the first part of this book— **the only change with this section will be using that information to identify when ovulation is happening!**

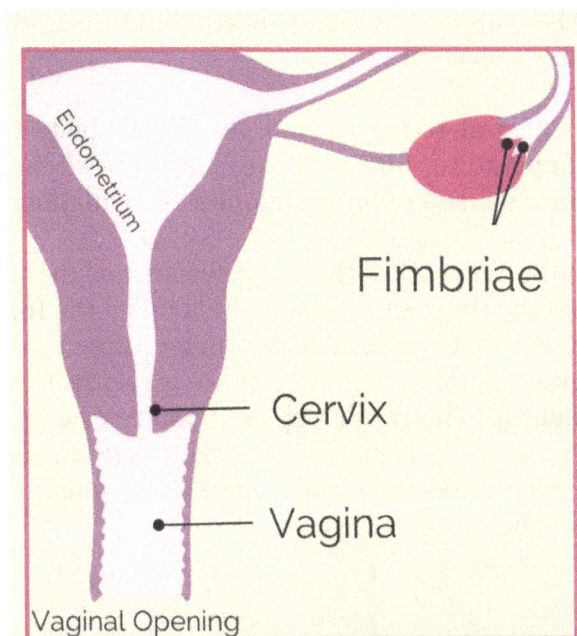

BASAL BODY TEMPERATURE: A NEW SIGN TO OBSERVE

Basal Body Temperature (BBT) is the measurement of your temperature first thing in the morning, after you've had a good sleep and before you get up. Prior to ovulation, your BBT is relatively low. After ovulation, your BBT is a little bit higher due to the presence of progesterone. If you are consistent about taking your temperature, you can verify that ovulation has happened simply by recording this slight shift in your resting temperature.

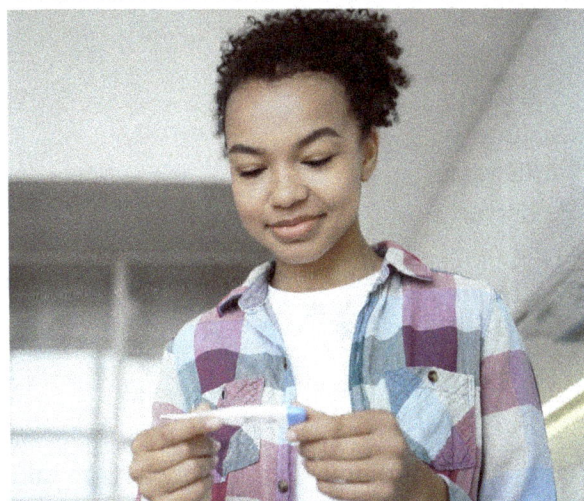

OTHER SIGNS

Fluid and temps are not the only signs our body gives us which can tell us about ovulation. Some women also track their hormones directly through simple urine tests, or observe physical changes in the position of the cervix. But in this guide, we will learn just how to start with fluid and temps, because they are the easiest and most helpful to learn when you are starting.

There is still a lot to discover about how our body "speaks" to us or gives us clues about all the invisible work it is doing! As our knowledge about menstrual cycles grows and our technology improves, it's possible we could develop lots of other ways to track ovulation that we don't even know about yet.

OBSERVING BBT
LEARNING A NEW SKILL

Observing your basal body temperature is different than just taking your temperature when you have a fever.

Instead of trying to find out if your body is fighting an infection and therefore above normal temperature, BBT is about measuring slight changes in your resting temperature which are the normal result of progesterone after ovulation.

In the first part of this book, we learned that the time following ovulation is called the **luteal phase** and the time before ovulation is called the **follicular phase.** During our menstrual cycle, we should expect that our basal body temperature in the follicular phase is relatively low, and our basal body temperature in the luteal phase is relatively high. But we're not talking about a huge shift: maybe about 0.5 (half) of a degree if you're observing temperatures in Fahrenheit or even just 0.2 (two tenths) of a degree if you are observing in Celsius. In this guide, we will focus on tracking temperatures in F, but I have some quick notes along the way which offer insights if you are temping in C!

Each dot represents a day of BBT. Note the lower values in follicular phase and higher values in luteal phase.

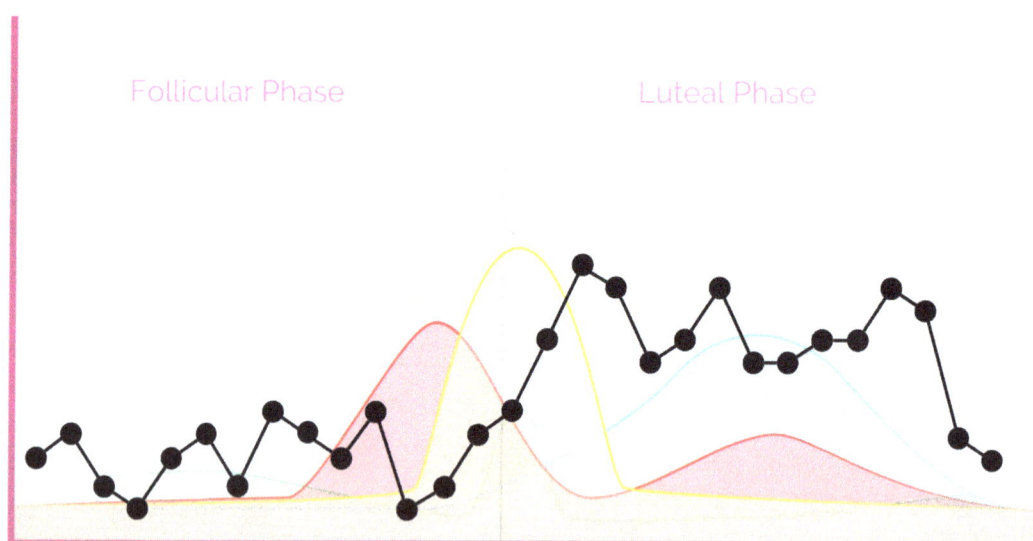

You may be thinking: "But I know how to take my temperature if I think I have a fever. How is BBT different? How do I capture my 'resting temperature'? What does that even mean?"

These are all great questions!
BBT is measured differently from regular temperatures in two ways:
1. it requires an additional level of accuracy in your actual thermometer, because we can be looking for some pretty small shifts!
2. you can only measure BBT after a period of rest, meaning you would usually check your temperature right when you wake up in the morning.

In order to meet these two important criteria for BBT, there are a few options you can consider. The first option is to go "classic" and just use an oral thermometer under your tongue, first thing in the morning when you wake up. The second option is to go more high tech and use a wearable thermometer. We'll talk about the pros and cons for both of those options in the following pages.

TEMP "CLASSIC": ORAL THERMOMETER

CHOOSING A THERMOMETER

To observe your basal body temperature, you can't use the same thermometer your family would use to check for fevers. For starters, you'll need to have your OWN thermometer which can be kept by your bed and used every day.

Secondly, you'll need a specific type of thermometer which is probably different from the one your family uses for fevers. You need **a basal body thermometer**, meaning that it has the accuracy you will need. A proper basal body thermometer will give you temperature readings accurate to the hundredths of a degree (two decimal points).

You don't have to get anything expensive or fancy, although it is possible to find many thermometers with lots of neat features. Some thermometers will have Bluetooth capability so they can sync directly to your phone for easy app charting. Others will save dozens of temperatures, offer quick read times, timers, and a backlit display for easy reading in the dark.

Do you need all of this? Nope!

All you need to look for is a BBT thermometer which allows you to recall at least one temperature, so you don't have to chart your results right away. This should only cost about $15-20 dollars and can get you a thermometer which will last a long time.

HOW TO TAKE YOUR TEMP

Keep your special BBT thermometer near your bed. You'll need to take your temperature **when you wake up,** before you get out of bed and before you do anything that might affect your temperature (like drink a glass of water).

Place the thermometer gently in your mouth, under your tongue (have your parent help you remember how to do this if needed). Close your mouth, and breathe through your nose while the thermometer does its reading. Some thermometers will beep every few seconds to let you know they are working; others will wait to beep until they are done taking the temperature.

To get the best, most accurate results, it's good to try to take your temperature at the same time each day; however, this isn't strictly required and I'll have some tips later in this guide if your temperature patterns seem a little jumpy.

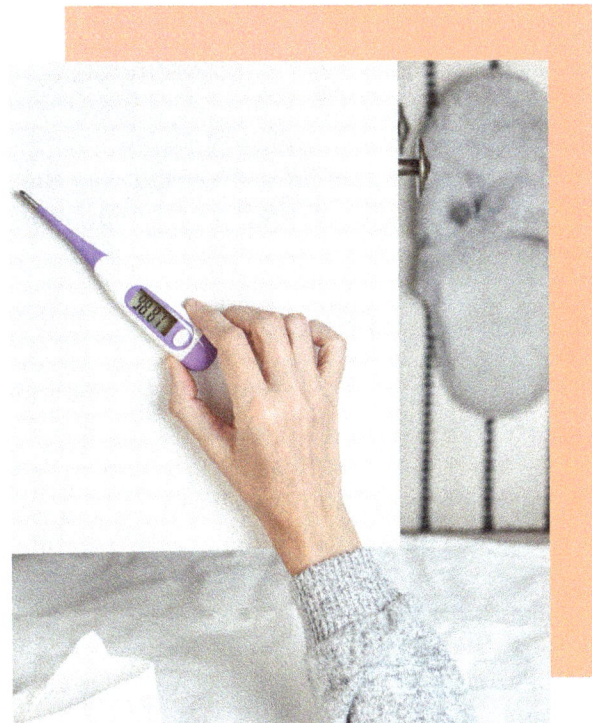

WEARABLE THERMOMETERS

CHOOSING A THERMOMETER

If you read the previous page, you may have noticed that getting the best accuracy with oral thermometers will require waking up around the same time each day. During the school year, this is probably something that most girls can do pretty easily, since our schedules are regular; but what about during summer? On break? On weekends? If your sleep schedules are irregular, it might still be possible to get accurate temperature data, or you might have a hard time getting accurate temps and may just not feel like it's worth the effort.

Because guess what? If you're thinking that charting takes a lot of effort- you're right! This is why I always tell girls (and reiterate again and again) that unless there's some sort of medical need, **you're never required to chart** your cycle for health! This is simply about learning to "read" your body and understand this very hidden aspect of how our female bodies work.

So, it's entirely possible that you might just say, "No thanks. I don't want to temp at all!"

Or maybe you'll think, "I want to get temperatures, but is there an easier way than waking up and taking my temperature orally?"

And the answer to that question is YES!

There are quite a few wearable devices that can monitor your temperature while you sleep. They may not be as accurate as an oral thermometer, and at the time I'm writing this guide, they don't have the research behind them to prove that they can find shifts in the same way we can with oral temps. But they might still be a good option to try! So here are some things to consider:

YOU ACTUALLY HAVE MANY DIFFERENT TEMPERATURES

When we think about Fahrenheit, a typical body temperature is somewhere around 98.6°, right? That's correct, if you're talking about oral temperatures.

But if you were to take your temperature in your ear, normal range is at least 0.5° higher, a little over 99° F.

If you take your temperature under your arm, normal is a little lower at about 98.1° F. Forehead scanners are similar.

And if we're looking at our skin temperature, depending on how far we are from the core of the body, a normal value can be anywhere from about 92-98° F, which is a HUGE range!

So, the first thing to understand and take into account with wearable thermometers is **what type of temperature** reading you are getting, and how accurate that might be relative to your core body temperature.

At this point, most wearables will give you readings from the skin temperature of your wrist or finger. Some others will measure temperatures under the arm (also called axillary temperature) which has a tighter studied range. Just be aware that it's normal to see different temperature ranges with these different tracking options, and that not all of them are likely to be as accurate as oral temps.

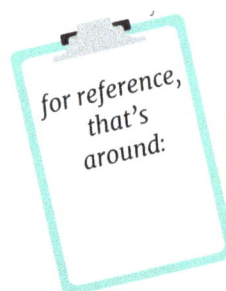

for reference, that's around:

ORAL- 37° C
EAR- 37.3° C
UNDER ARM- 36.7° C
SKIN- 33-37° C

A NOTE ABOUT TECH...

In the first part of this guide, we learned about some of the pros and cons to utilizing apps for charting. It's worth taking some time to make similar comments about the pros and cons of using high tech temperature tracking devices, whether that's an oral thermometer which links via Bluetooth to your phone, or a wearable device that syncs data in other ways.

Technology is great when it can make certain tasks easier and more straightforward! But "femtech" (that is, technology geared towards tracking women's cycles) is a multi-billion dollar industry. Some companies really do care a lot about empowering women and making this valuable information accessible. But other companies see this as a way to make some quick money, and they are therefore more interested in selling their product than in teaching you how to observe and understand your own body.

So if you are thinking of getting a nice, high-tech temping device, here are some things you and your parents should probably talk about and consider:

- **Does this device try to interpret my data for me? Or does it give me the freedom to interpret data and learn things on my own?** This is REALLY important for teens, because interpretive or predictive algorithms are not built for times (like the years of puberty) where it's totally normal for cycles to be more irregular. Interpretive features may be inaccurate, or create unnecessary worry. Plus, they don't actually empower YOU to be literate about your body. And guess who has an interest in making you dependent upon their interpretive technology? Companies that want to keep selling you their technology.
- **What do these companies do with my data?** Do they sell it to other companies? Do they use my data for research? Do they keep it private? How do I feel about that?
- **Do I have to pay to get data that the device could be tracking for free?** This is a big pet peeve of mine, because some devices are capable of tracking a LOT of health information, but they don't include temperature as part of their free information. Some companies will require you to pay an additional subscription to get temperature data. So just be sure you know the full cost before investing in a device.

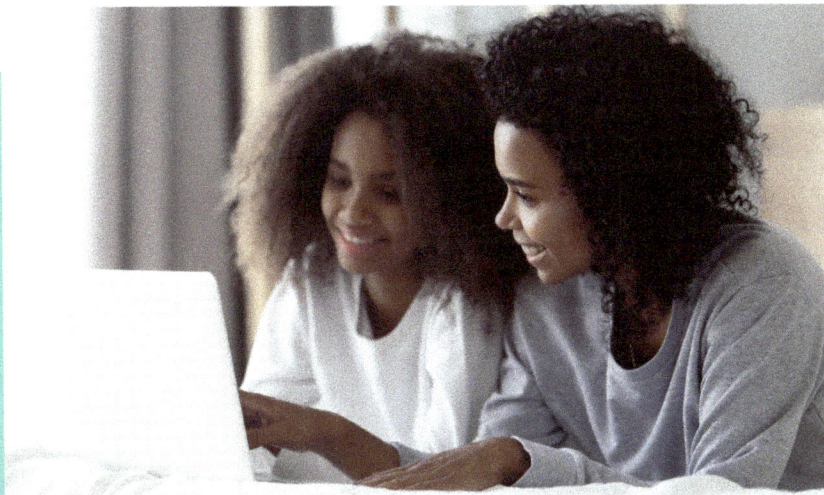

> **SUMMARY:**
> Take time to research any devices you are interested in using for cycle tracking, to make sure the thermometer is suitable for your situation, goals and preferences!

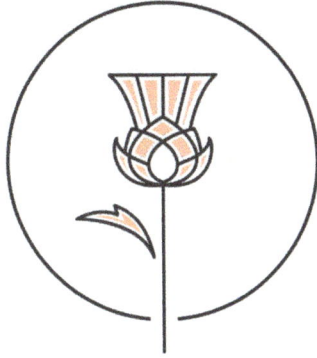

FINDING OVULATION
ON A CHART

HOW TO CHART TEMPERATURES

At the beginning of this guide, you learned about two different styles of chart: a wheel chart and a linear chart. Both of them contained the same information, even though some of the formatting was different. But neither of them had an option for temperatures, which we just learned about in the previous section.

So, in order to add temperatures to our charts, we're going to need to expand that linear chart to contain a full graph, like this:

Date																																												
Day of Cycle	1	2	3	4	5	6	7	8	9	10	11	12	13	14	15	16	17	18	19	20	21	22	23	24	25	26	27	28	29	30	31	32	33	34	35	36	37	38	39	40	41	42	43	44	45

Year _____ — temperature graph ranging from 98.9° down to 97.0°

Cycle # _____ — temperature graph ranging from 97.9° down to 96.0°

Day of Cycle	1	2	3	4	5	6	7	8	9	10	11	12	13	14	15	16	17	18	19	20	21	22	23	24	25	26	27	28	29	30	31	32	33	34	35	36	37	38	39	40	41	42	43	44	45
Period & Fluid																																													
Fluid Notations																																													
Period Pain?																																													
My Mood																																													

KEY

Fluid Notations
L= Light Flow   M= Moderate Flow   H = Heavy Flow

Period & Fluid
Red = flow of blood   Dots = spotting   Gray = dry, no fluid
Yellow = moist/sticky, pasty, creamy, slightly stretchy fluid
Teal = slippery/wet, clear, stretchy, slippery, watery fluid

Period Pain
0 = no pain
1 = a little uncomfortable
2 = medium amount of discomfort
3 = pain interferes with my day

Mood
+ = Happy
☆ = Neutral
-- = Sad
@ = Stressed
# = Angry

My Cycles This Past Year

Shortest Cycle _____   Longest Cycle _____

Shortest Period _____   Longest Period _____

The bottom information for periods, fluid notations, and other tracking options all stays the same, but now we've added a graph from 96.0-98.9° F which will help us track temperatures. While cervical fluid is charted at the end of the day (because you have to gather all of your observations from the day!), temperature can either be charted first thing in the morning or at the same time you chart your fluid at the end of the day—as long as you have a thermometer which can store a temperature reading for you to pull up later!

Note also there's now a place to keep track of your cycle "stats," which is helpful for observing patterns. It's just a record of key pieces of information from the past year: shortest and longest cycle lengths, with shortest and longest periods.

HOW TO CHART TEMPERATURES

Even though your thermometer is accurate to two decimal points, we will only chart to one decimal point (to the tenths). You could round if you prefer, but **the easiest way to do this is to just cut off the last number (called truncating)!** So that's what we'll do in our sample charts:

- If your thermometer reads 97.83°, then put a dot at 97.8 on the chart.
- If your thermometer reads 97.88°, then put a dot at 97.8 on the chart.

Each day, connect your new dot to the day before it, and you'll make a nice graph!

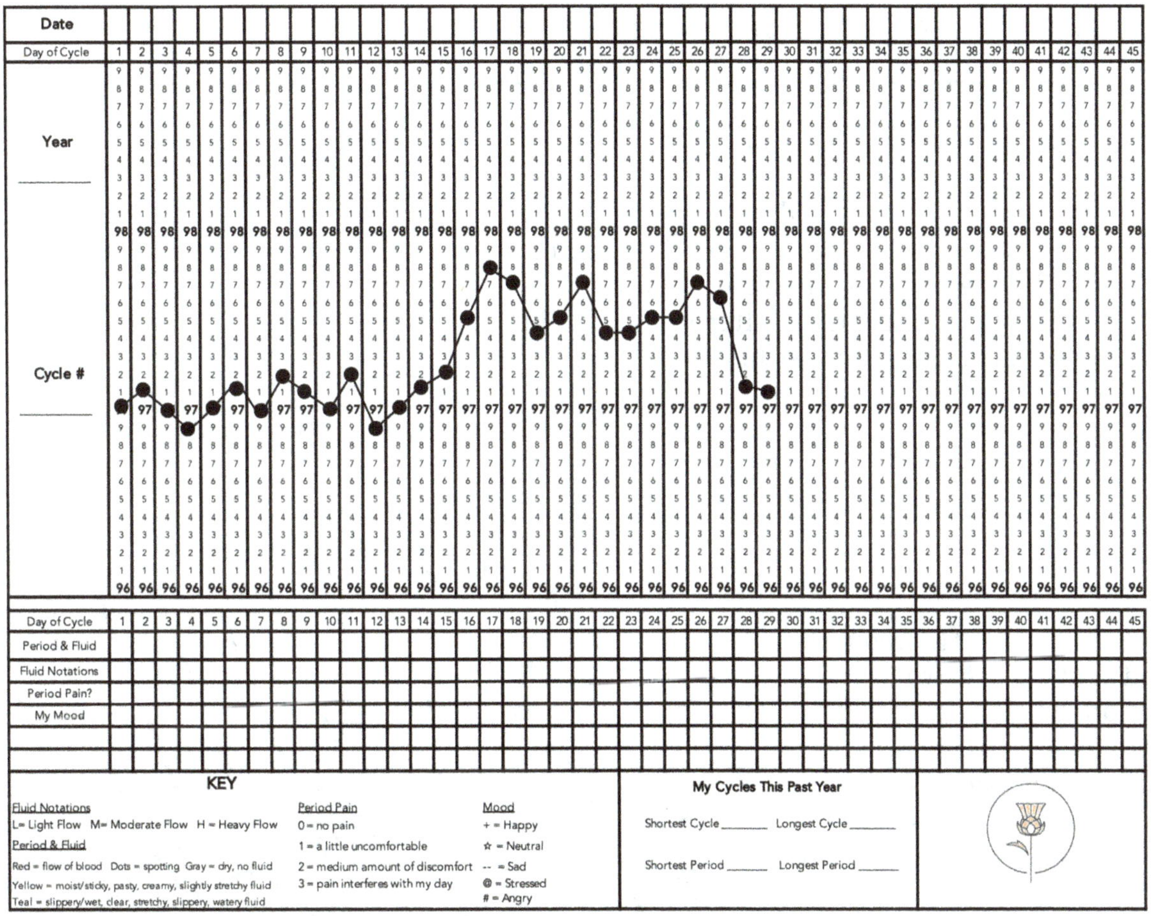

Date
Day of Cycle
Year
Cycle #
Day of Cycle
Period & Fluid
Fluid Notations
Period Pain?
My Mood
KEY
Fluid Notations
L= Light Flow M= Moderate Flow H = Heavy Flow
Period & Fluid
Red = flow of blood Dots = spotting Gray = dry, no fluid
Yellow = moist/sticky, pasty, creamy, slightly stretchy fluid
Teal = slippery/wet, clear, stretchy, slippery, watery fluid
Period Pain
0 = no pain
1 = a little uncomfortable
2 = medium amount of discomfort
3 = pain interferes with my day
Mood
+ = Happy
☆ = Neutral
-- = Sad
@ = Stressed
# = Angry
My Cycles This Past Year
Shortest Cycle ____ Longest Cycle ____
Shortest Period ____ Longest Period ____

Note that if you have a chart for tracking temperatures in Celsius, you will NOT be charting to the tenth of a degree! Instead you will be **charting to the nearest 0.05 of a degree,** meaning that all your numbers will end either with a 5 or a 0. This will require a little bit of rounding!

Example Temp	**Rounds To**
37.10	**37.10**
36.09	**37.10**
36.08	**37.10**
36.07	**36.05**
36.06	**36.05**
36.05	**36.05**
36.04	**36.05**
36.03	**36.05**
36.02	**36.00**
36.01	**36.00**
36.00	**36.00**

FINDING OVULATION
USING FLUID + TEMPERATURES

Now that you know how to chart cervical fluid and BBT which are two signs of ovulation, let's talk about how to use that information! We'll be looking for signs which tell us that ovulation has passed, so we have the option of doing two different calculations:

1) IDENTIFY FLUID PEAK DAY

2) IDENTIFY A TEMP SHIFT

You can do these together, or choose to do just one.

IDENTIFYING THE FLUID PEAK DAY:

Around ovulation time, your body will make the TEAL category of fluid, so we'll check to see when it stops making this fluid to let us know that ovulation has likely passed. The **Fluid Peak Day** is the last day of fluid recorded with a TEAL color block, followed by 4 consecutive NOT teal days. Fluid Peak Day can only be identified after it occurs. Fluid observations after Fluid Peak Day may be YELLOW or GRAY observations—this is fine!

Using the "Fluid Notations" line on your chart, mark Fluid Peak Day with a STAR and number the four consecutive days after Fluid Peak Day

These five days of TEAL could be called a **fluid patch,** which is a common thing to see leading up to ovulation. However, you may not get a clear patch like this: instead you could see a mixed pattern like: G, Y, T, T, Y, T, Y, T

What you're really looking for to identify Fluid Peak Day is a TEAL followed by four consecutive not-TEALs. This will tell you that ovulation has **likely** passed.

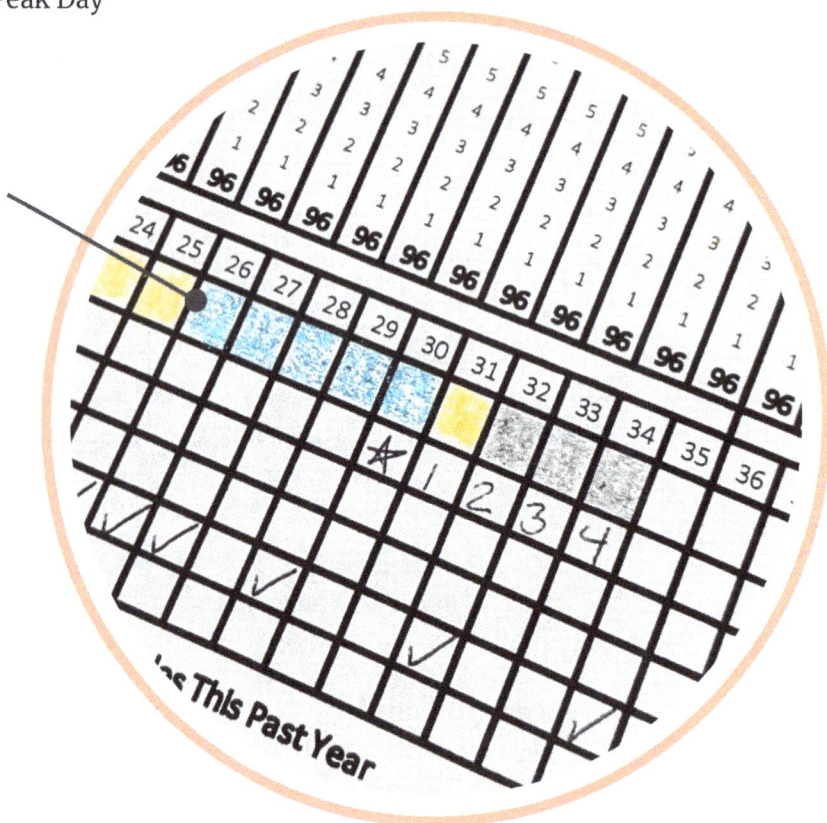

FINDING OVULATION
USING FLUID + TEMPERATURES

IDENTIFYING A TEMPERATURE SHIFT

Another thing we can look for to tell us that ovulation has occurred is a temperature shift. Cervical fluid tells us when ovulation is *about to happen* because it responds mostly to estrogen, which is the dominant hormone before ovulation. A **temperature shift tells us that ovulation has already happened, because it responds to progesterone**—the dominant hormone after ovulation.

As you are learning how to identify a temperature shift, I find that it's easiest to begin doing this calculation at the END of a cycle, after the full chart is already complete. So when you start a new period bleed, you can look back on the previous chart and see where ovulation was confirmed (if at all!). As you get used to doing the calculation, you'll be able to see your shifts happening in real time, which can give you some great information on where you are, currently, with your cycle.

There are actually a lot of different ways researchers have found to calculate temperature shifts. The method we will learn how to do has three steps:

- **FIRST:** find 4 temps higher than the previous 6
- **SECOND:** calculate your **Coverline**
- **THIRD:** look for 4 temps over the Coverline

It's important to take these steps one at a time!

First Step:

Go day by day across the chart and identify **four consecutive temperatures** which, as a set, are higher than the six temperatures that come right before them. This tells you that progesterone is probably present and working hard.

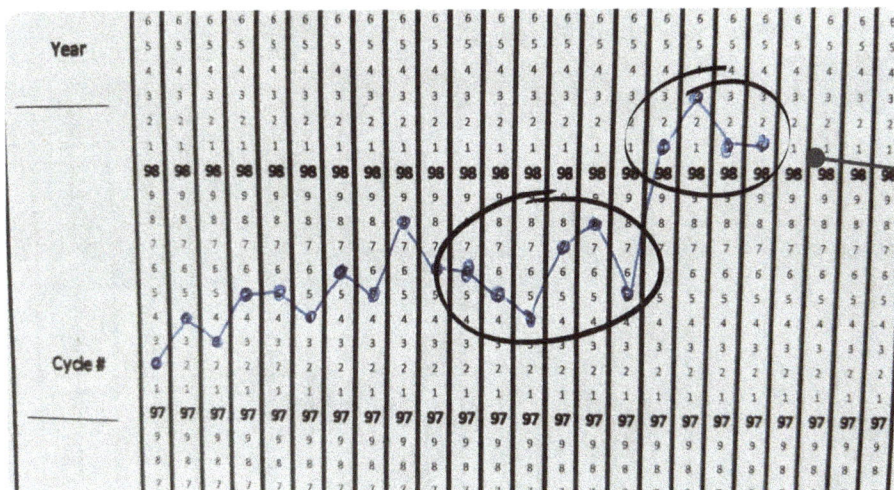

These four temperatures are higher than the six which come before them.

Note: it doesn't matter if they are higher than each other! It only matters that they, as a group, are higher than the 6 days before.

FINDING OVULATION
USING FLUID + TEMPERATURES

Second Step:

Locate the highest temperature of the six low temperatures.
Draw a line across the chart 1/10th of a degree above this highest temperature. This is your
Coverline and it is the dividing line between your low and your high temps.

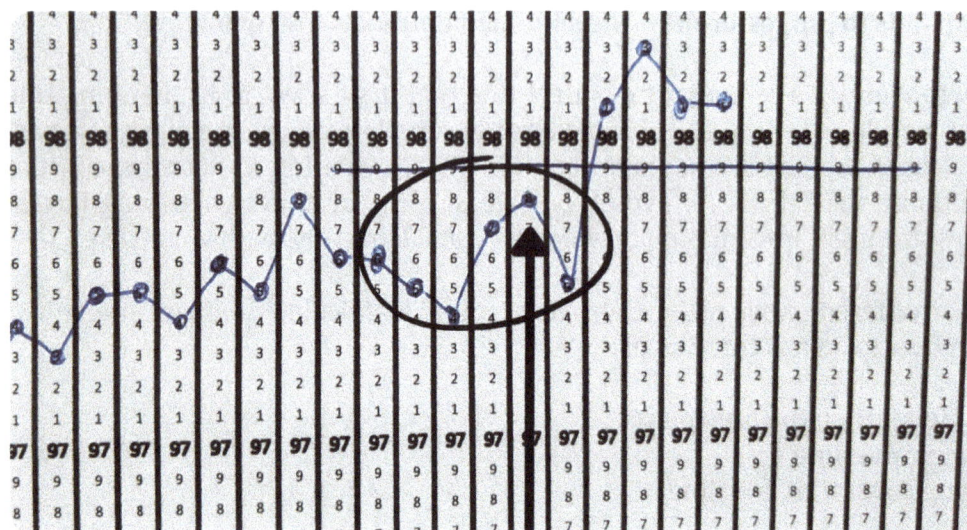

The highest temp of the low 6 was at 97.8, so your Coverline goes right at 97.9°.

Note: when you are setting the Coverline, don't worry if there are temperatures earlier in your chart that might be on or above the line. You only need to look at the 6 temps which are right before your 4 high ones.

Third Step:

Number the first four temperatures above the line. Temps which are resting on the line don't count since they don't show us that progesterone is strong enough yet, but once you have four temps above the Coverline, this confirms for you that ovulation has passed!

Once you identify a shift, watch for a temp that drops below your Coverline about 1-2 weeks later. Not all girls see this, but if you do, it could be a signal that your period will start very soon!

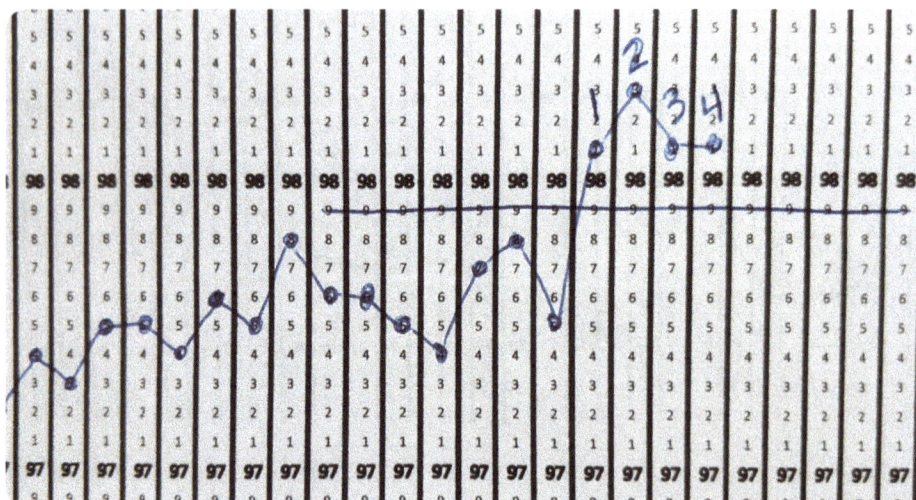

FINDING OVULATION
USING FLUID + TEMPERATURES

Helpful hint:
Take it just a day at a time

Each day, it's an interesting thing to just ask yourself: **is today's temperature higher than the six before it?** In most cases, that answer will be simple: NO!

But sometimes, the answer will be YES! In which case, you shouldn't assume that you're seeing a temperature shift necessarily. Temperatures can just go up and down sometimes, and that's normal.

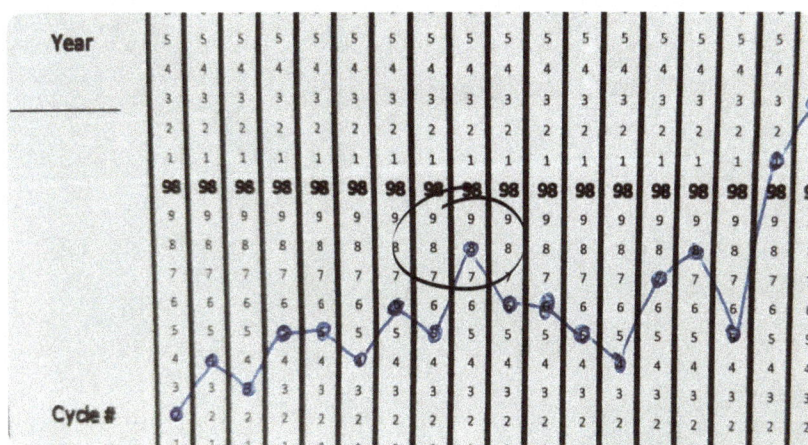

For example: When you get this temperature here at 98.8, you might think a shift is starting because it is higher than the 6 before it! But you know not to assume anything, so you simply make a mental note to keep track of whether the next 3 days are also higher than the previous 6... which, in this case does not happen.

So you just keep charting! And then in a few days you end up finding the shift we just calculated in the previous pages, with a Coverline above that temp at 97.9.°

What about Celsius?

The calculations for finding a shift in Celsius are pretty similar to finding a shift in F, but you'd need a special chart with those temperature markings. Most apps have options for either F or C, so electronic charting may be your preference in that case, since it might be more comfortable than learning a new temperature scale.

If you are going to find a shift with Celsius, you'll still follow the basics of the three steps we just went through; but instead of going up a tenth of a degree (0.1), you can approximate the Coverline calculation by going up 5 hundredths (0.05) of a degree.

The calculation is the same one we learned for F: once you have four temperatures above that line, it's a good sign that progesterone is likely working and ovulation has likely passed.

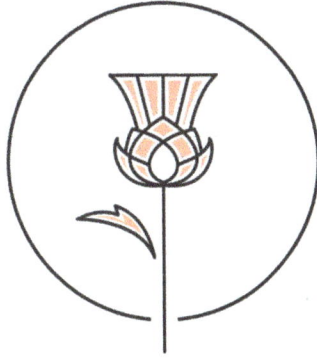

PRACTICE CHARTS
AND TIPS

TRYING OUT WHAT YOU KNOW

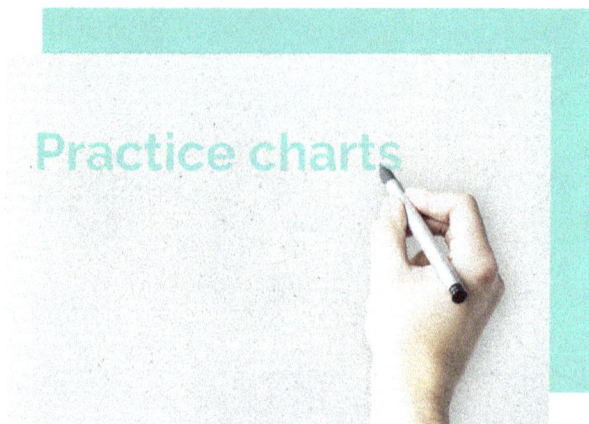

Practice charts

You've now learned how to look for ovulation in a cycle, and you know why this might be important.

In this next section, we'll do a few practice charts to help you feel confident identifying that ovulation has passed, but before we do that, a few quick notes:

YOUR CHARTS WILL PROBABLY NOT LOOK LIKE THE SAMPLES

And that is okay. Charting in real life is harder than putting together a sample chart. Your sleep may get disturbed, you might get sick, or any number of things may happen which make your charts harder to interpret. When this happens, don't worry! I'll reiterate what was said earlier: if your charts ever lead you to think negatively about yourself, then it is no longer fulfilling its function and you should feel free to let it go!

TWO (OR MORE!) FLUID PEAK DAYS

If you have a delayed ovulation, you might have more than one patch of TEAL type fluid as your estrogen ebbs and flows. This is perfectly normal—and it's why adding temperatures to confirm that ovulation has definitely passed is a great combination.

YOUR COVERLINES MONTH-TO-MONTH

As long as you are using the same thermometer, you might notice that your Coverline is often in a consistent place, within a few tenths of a degree each month. Or not. It can just depend! So don't worry if it's always the same, or if it varies a lot! Either is fine.

YOU CAN'T PINPOINT THE EXACT DAY OF OVULATION

We've said it before, but we'll say it again, because it's important to keep this in mind! You have learned rules which help you identify that ovulation **has already passed**, but without doing bloodwork or going in for an ultrasound every day, it's impossible to tell exactly which day you ovulated. Cervical fluid will change within a few days of ovulation. Temps will rise within a couple days of ovulation. So don't sweat trying to pinpoint the exact day.

This also means that you won't know **exactly** how long your luteal phase is, since you can't know the exact day you ovulated. But you may notice patterns—you may notice a consistent amount of days your temperature stays high before your next bleed starts, or a consistent number of days after your fluid peak. Or you'll be within a couple of days each time. Keep an eye out for these patterns, because they are unique to you!

SIGNS THAT DON'T LINE UP

Because cervical fluid and temps can respond to hormones within a few days of ovulation, they might not always line up perfectly! You may reach Peak + 4 with fluid, but only have 2 high temps. Or you may have 4 high temps and still have a couple days of TEAL type fluid afterwards. This is fine! Remember: a menstrual cycle is a complicated symphony of hormones.

Practice Chart #1

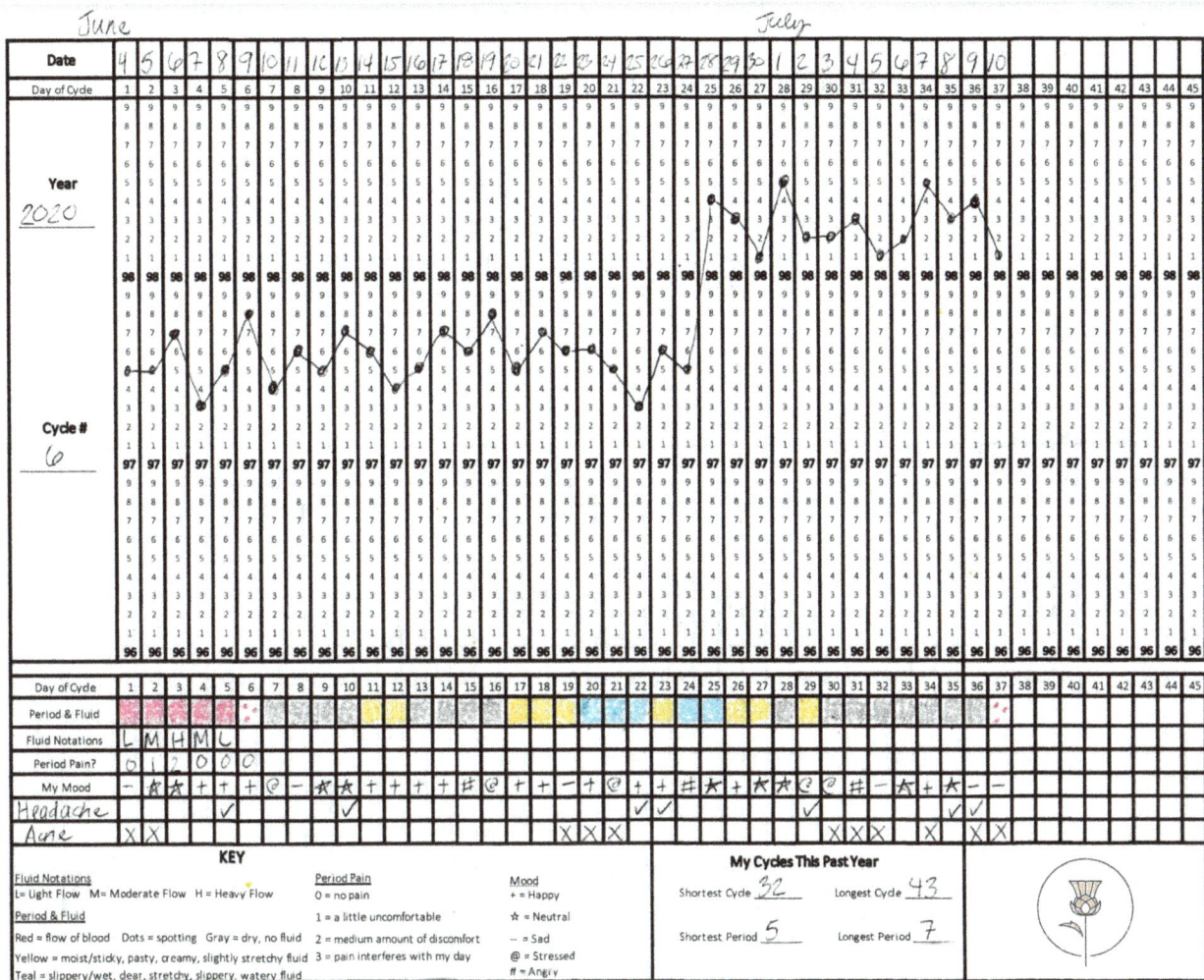

The chart shows handwritten months "June" and "July" across the top, with a basal body temperature tracking grid for Year 2020, Cycle #6.

KEY

Fluid Notations
L= Light Flow   M= Moderate Flow   H = Heavy Flow

Period & Fluid
Red = flow of blood   Dots = spotting   Gray = dry, no fluid
Yellow = moist/sticky, pasty, creamy, slightly stretchy fluid
Teal = slippery/wet, clear, stretchy, slippery, watery fluid

Period Pain
0 = no pain
1 = a little uncomfortable
2 = medium amount of discomfort
3 = pain interferes with my day

Mood
+ = Happy
☆ = Neutral
-- = Sad
@ = Stressed
# = Angry

My Cycles This Past Year
Shortest Cycle 32   Longest Cycle 43
Shortest Period 5   Longest Period 7

To look for ovulation, we will try to identify two things:

1) Fluid Peak Day +4
2) 4 days of Temperature Shift

Fluid peak is identified by looking for a TEAL that is followed by four days of not teal, meaning either YELLOW or GRAY. On Day 25 of this cycle, you can see that she has a TEAL observation and then that is followed by YELLOW on Day 26, YELLOW on Day 27, GRAY on Day 28, and YELLOW again on Day 29. So by Day 29 she thinks, "Aha! Maybe my cervical fluid pattern is telling me that ovulation has passed for this cycle!"

She could choose to go ahead and mark her Fluid Peak in the line for "Fluid Notations" at that point, or she can just wait until she starts her next bleed to mark up the current chart. Either approach is fine! But now let's look at how she'd find ovulation with her temperatures:

Practice Chart #1

When we look at this chart example here, we're looking at a completed chart at the end of a cycle. I highly recommend waiting until the end of a menstrual cycle to do the temperature calculation whe you are first learning, because it can be much easier to see shifts when the cycle is complete than it is to find shifts as they are happening.

If you just look at this chart, you can see that there's a long portion at the beginning of the cycle where temperatures are all below 98°. And there's a portion of the chart where it's easy to see that the temps are all over 98°! So a shift has definitely happened and we have a pretty good sense that it happened starting on Day 25. But let's go ahead and do the different steps of the temperature calculation to make sure!

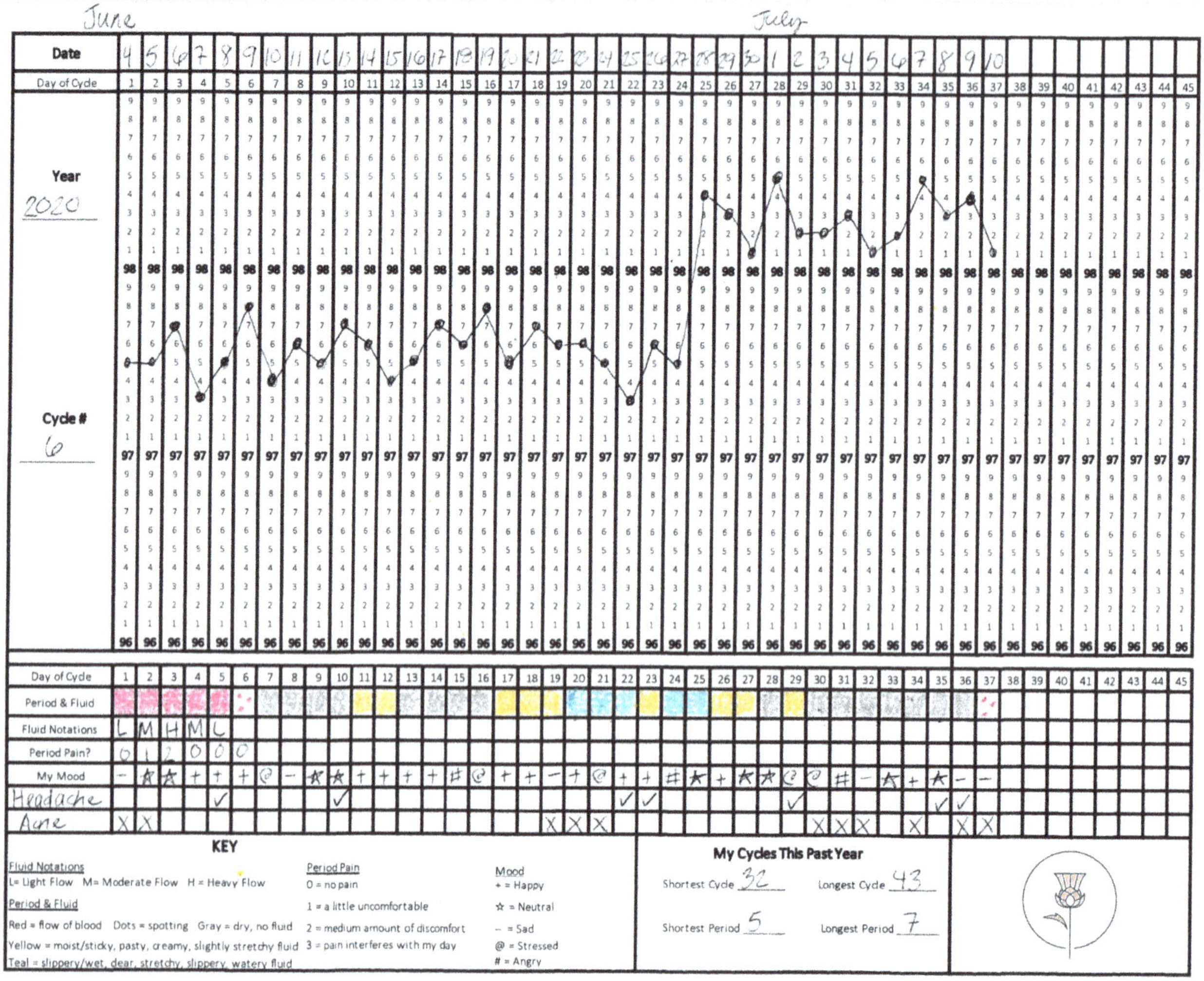

June
July
Date
Day of Cycle
Year
2020
Cycle #
6
Period & Fluid
Fluid Notations
Period Pain?
My Mood
Headache
Acne
KEY
Fluid Notations
L= Light Flow M= Moderate Flow H = Heavy Flow
Period & Fluid
Red = flow of blood Dots = spotting Gray = dry, no fluid
Yellow = moist/sticky, pasty, creamy, slightly stretchy fluid
Teal = slippery/wet, clear, stretchy, slippery, watery fluid
Period Pain
0 = no pain
1 = a little uncomfortable
2 = medium amount of discomfort
3 = pain interferes with my day
Mood
+ = Happy
☆ = Neutral
– = Sad
@ = Stressed
# = Angry
My Cycles This Past Year
Shortest Cycle 32
Longest Cycle 43
Shortest Period 5
Longest Period 7

Practice Chart #1

To make this easier to do, we'll just zoom in on the temperature part of the graph, looking specifically at the days around Day 25, when we suspect the shift happened:

First Step:

Go day by day across the chart and identify **four consecutive temperatures** which, as a set, are higher than the six temperatures that come right before them. This tells you that progesterone is working hard!

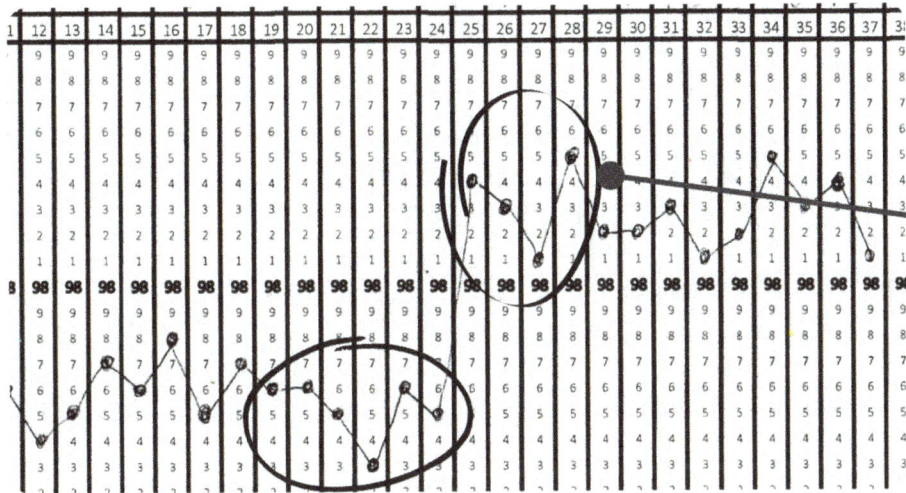

These four temperatures on Days 25, 26, 27, and 28 are higher than the six which come before them.

Second Step:

Locate the highest temperature of the six low temperatures.
Draw a line across the chart 1/10th of a degree above this highest temperature. This is your **Coverline** and it is the dividing line between your low and your high temps.

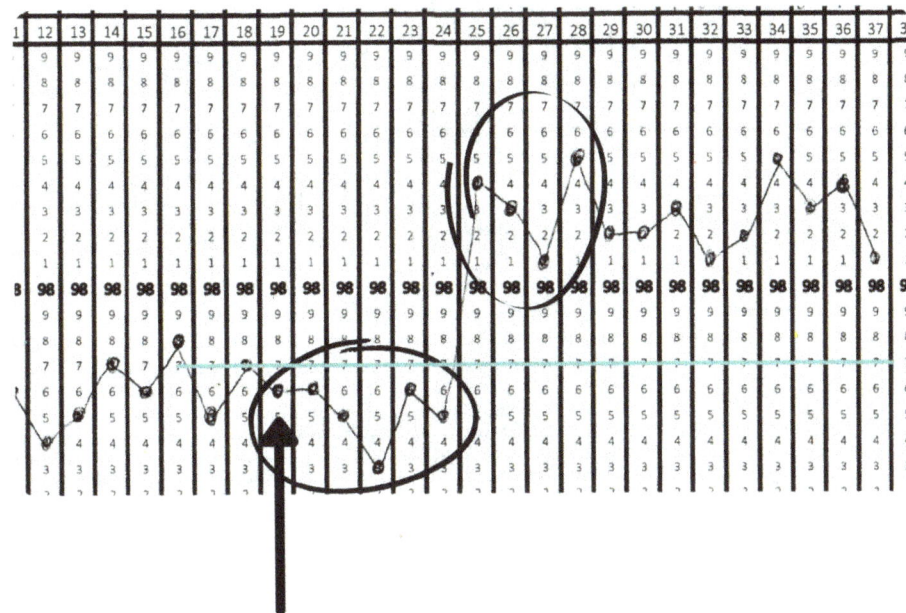

There were a few recordings of 97.6° in this set of numbers before the shift. This is the highest value within that set (it's okay if you had temps higher than that earlier!), so the Coverline goes right at 97.7°.

Practice Chart #1

Third Step:

Number the first four temperatures above the line. This confirms for you that ovulation has passed!

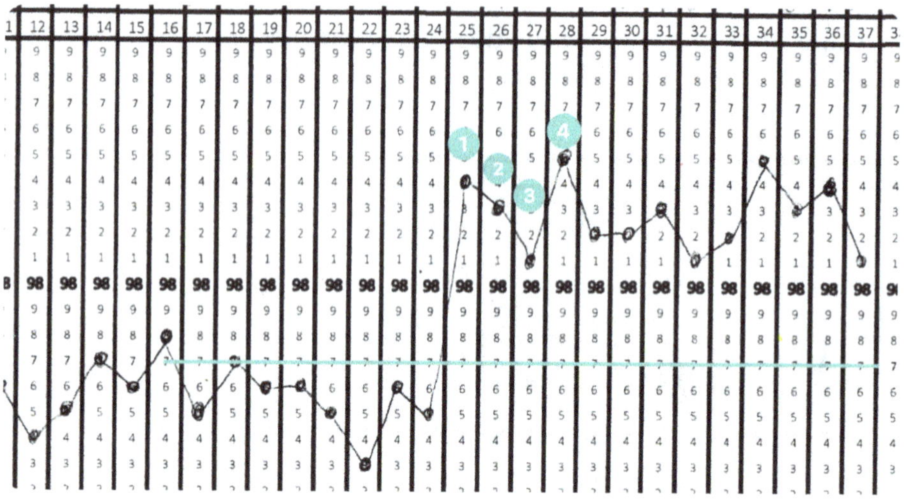

So this chart shows a **Fluid Peak day** and **Temp Shift** both starting at **Day 25! Ovulation confirmed.**

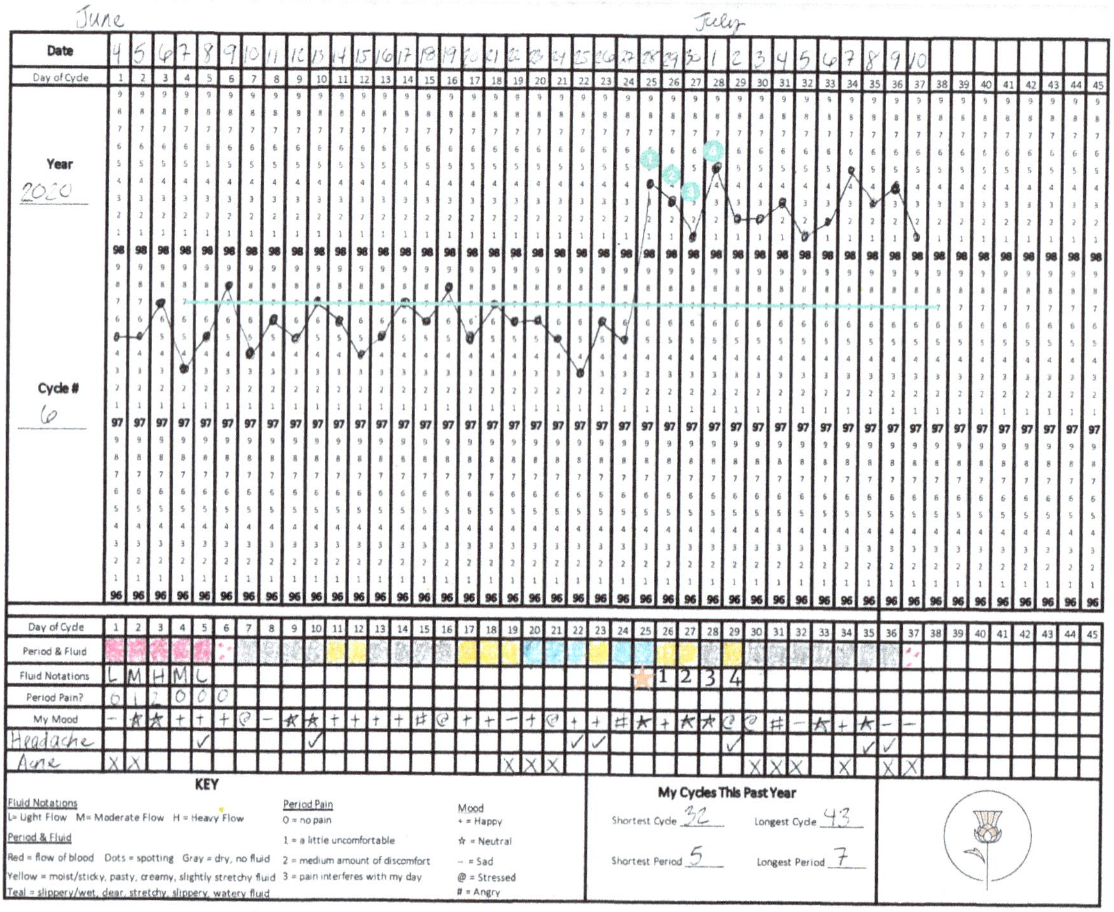
June
July
Date
Day of Cycle
Year
2020
Cycle #
6
Period & Fluid
Fluid Notations
Period Pain?
My Mood
Headache
Acne
KEY
Fluid Notations
L= Light Flow M= Moderate Flow H = Heavy Flow
Period & Fluid
Red = flow of blood Dots = spotting Gray = dry, no fluid
Yellow = moist/sticky, pasty, creamy, slightly stretchy fluid
Teal = slippery/wet, clear, stretchy, slippery, watery fluid
Period Pain
0 = no pain
1 = a little uncomfortable
2 = medium amount of discomfort
3 = pain interferes with my day
Mood
+ = Happy
☆ = Neutral
– = Sad
@ = Stressed
# = Angry
My Cycles This Past Year
Shortest Cycle 32
Longest Cycle 43
Shortest Period 5
Longest Period 7

Practice Chart #1

Here's the same chart in the Read Your Body app, put together with custom fluid coloring and other categories.

Read Your Body allows you to manually input the Coverline and identify peak days.

To mark Peak Day on your chart, go to the Fluid section and click "Interpretation" > Peak day. Four days later, you can then mark "Count after peak is complete"

To set a Coverline for your temps, go to the 'Chart' view and tap the icon in the top right that looks like a pencil. This will let you manually enter where your Coverline can go. Then, in the Temperature section, click on "Interpretation" and you can mark either "Temp rise starts today" or "Temp rise is confirmed" when those apply!

Practice Chart #2

OCTOBER　　　　　　　　　　　　　　　　NOVEMBER

Date	7	8	9	10	11	12	13	14	15	16	17	18	19	20	21	22	23	24	25	26	27	28	29	30	31	1	2	3	4	5	6	7	8	9											
Day of Cycle	1	2	3	4	5	6	7	8	9	10	11	12	13	14	15	16	17	18	19	20	21	22	23	24	25	26	27	28	29	30	31	32	33	34	35	36	37	38	39	40	41	42	43	44	45

Year 2020　　Cycle # 10

Day of Cycle	1	2	3	4	5	6	7	8	9	10	11	12	13	14	15	16	17	18	19	20	21	22	23	24	25	26	27	28	29	30	31	32	33	34	35	36	37	38	39	40	41	42	43	44	45
Period & Fluid																																													
Fluid Notations	H	H	M	M	L																																								
Period Pain?	3	1	1	0	0																																								
My Mood																																													
Water	✓	✓	✓		✓	✓		✓			✓			✓		✓			✓	✓		✓		✓	✓	✓	✓																		

KEY

Fluid Notations
L = Light Flow　M = Moderate Flow　H = Heavy Flow

Period & Fluid
Red = flow of blood　Dots = spotting　Gray = dry, no fluid
Yellow = moist/sticky, pasty, creamy, slightly stretchy fluid
Teal = slippery/wet, clear, stretchy, slippery, watery fluid

Period Pain
0 = no pain
1 = a little uncomfortable
2 = medium amount of discomfort
3 = pain interferes with my day

Mood
+ = Happy
☆ = Neutral
⌣ = Sad
@ = Stressed
# = Angry

My Cycles This Past Year
Shortest Cycle 29　　Longest Cycle 39
Shortest Period 4　　Longest Period 6

To look for ovulation, we will try to identify two things:

1) Fluid Peak Day +4
2) 4 days of Temperature Shift

We can see that Day 24 of this cycle is a TEAL fluid day, followed by four days of YELLOW. So Fluid Peak Day can be marked as Day 24.

But what about the temperatures? There are a few missing data points here, which is pretty normal. Remember, charting isn't always going to be perfect and that's alright. But the question is whether we have enough information to calculate a shift.

If you are just looking at these patterns, you can see that temperatures in the first part of the cycle are lower and temperatures after that Fluid Peak Day are a little bit higher, closer to 98°. Let's see if we can apply the steps to find a shift:

Practice Chart #2

First Step:

Go day by day across the chart and identify **four consecutive temperatures** which, as a set, are higher than the temperatures in the six days that come right before them. This tells you that progesterone is probably working hard!

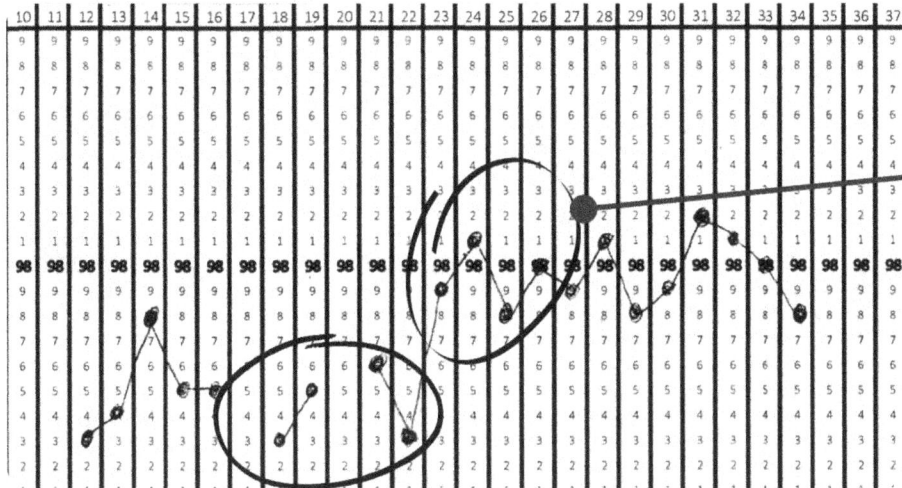

These four temperatures on Days 23, 24, 25 and 26 look like they could be higher than the six which come before them, but there are two missing days, so it's hard to be sure.

Technically it's just too much missing data to be one hundred percent confident, but we can see that all the rest of the temperatures following Day 26 were in the same sort of range, indicating a shift has happened. So in this case, we could approximate a Coverline just by using the data points we do have.

Second Step:

Locate the highest temperature of the six low temperatures.
Draw a line across the chart 1/10th of a degree above this highest temperature. This is your **Coverline** and it is the dividing line between your low and your high temps.

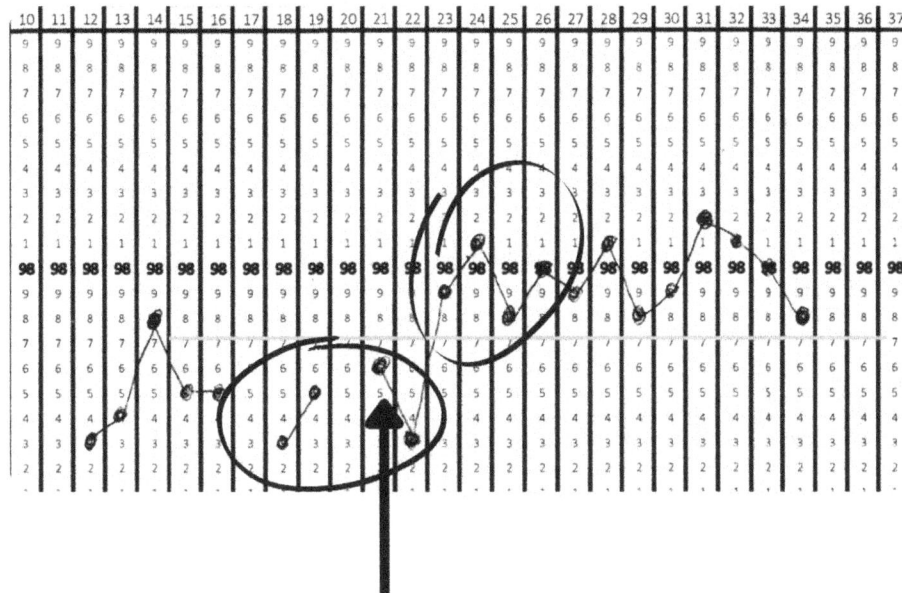

The highest recorded value we have in the six days before the shift is a 97.6°, so we can set an approximate Coverline at 97.7°.

-55-

Practice Chart #2

Third Step:

Number the first four temperatures above the line. This confirms for you that ovulation has passed!

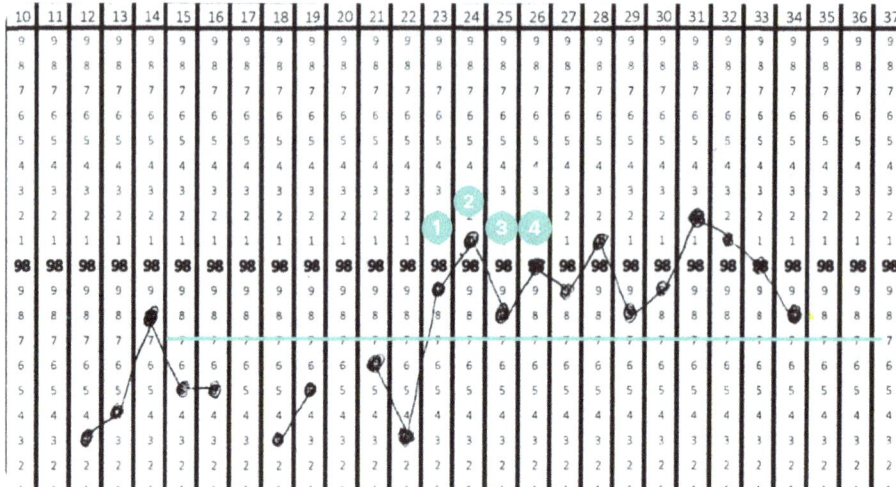

So this chart shows a **Fluid Peak Day** on Day 24 and a **Temp Shift** starting (we think!) on Day 23. **Ovulation is very likely confirmed.**

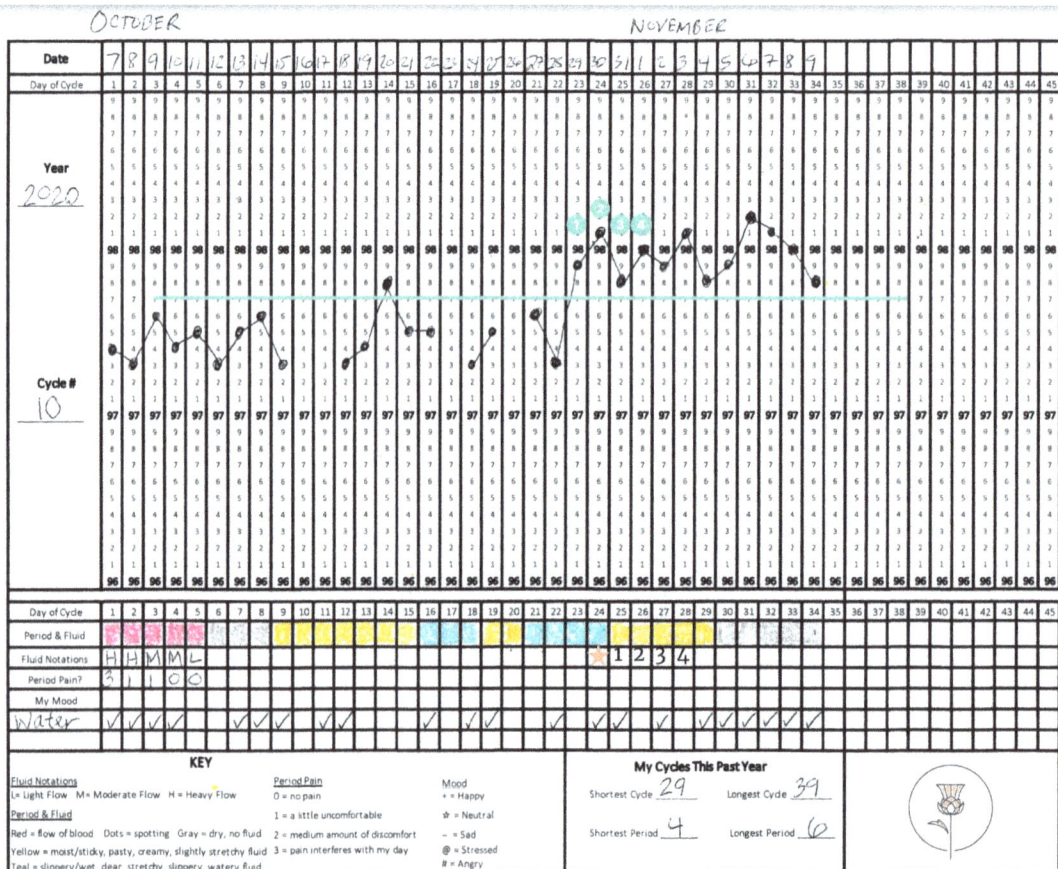

KEY

-56-

Practice Chart #3

Day of Cycle	1	2	3	4	5	6	7	8	9	10	11	12	13	14	15	16	17	18	19	20	21	22	23	24	25	26	27	28	29	30	31	32	33	34	35	36	37	38	39	40	41	42	43	44	45
Period & Fluid																																													
Fluid Notations	L	H	H	H	M	L	L																																						
Period Pain?																																													
My Mood																																													
Exercise																																													

KEY

Fluid Notations
L = Light Flow   M = Moderate Flow   H = Heavy Flow

Period & Fluid
Red = flow of blood   Dots = spotting   Gray = dry, no fluid
Yellow = moist/sticky, pasty, creamy, slightly stretchy fluid
Teal = slippery/wet, clear, stretchy, slippery, watery fluid

Period Pain
0 = no pain
1 = a little uncomfortable
2 = medium amount of discomfort
3 = pain interferes with my day

Mood
+ = Happy
☆ = Neutral
– = Sad
@ = Stressed
# = Angry

My Cycles This Past Year
Shortest Cycle 35   Longest Cycle 45
Shortest Period 6   Longest Period 8

Take note: there are no temperatures on this chart. Advanced charting to look for signs of ovulation can easily be done with just fluid observations. **Remember: what you chart is up to you!**

To look for ovulation, we will try to identify:

Fluid Peak Day +4

On this chart, we see that Day 30 is a TEAL day followed by a YELLOW, then three GRAY days. So all she would need to do with this chart is mark Day 30 as her Fluid Peak Day!

Day of Cycle	1	2	3	4	5	6	7	8	9	10	11	12	13	14	15	16	17	18	19	20	21	22	23	24	25	26	27	28	29	30	31	32	33	34	35	36	37	38	39	40	41	42	43	44	45
Period & Fluid																																													
Fluid Notations	L	H	H	H	M	L	L																							☆	1	2	3	4											
Period Pain?																																													
My Mood																																													
Exercise																																													

KEY

Fluid Notations
L = Light Flow   M = Moderate Flow   H = Heavy Flow

Period & Fluid
Red = flow of blood   Dots = spotting   Gray = dry, no fluid
Yellow = moist/sticky, pasty, creamy, slightly stretchy fluid
Teal = slippery/wet, clear, stretchy, slippery, watery fluid

Period Pain
0 = no pain
1 = a little uncomfortable
2 = medium amount of discomfort
3 = pain interferes with my day

Mood
+ = Happy
☆ = Neutral
– = Sad
@ = Stressed
# = Angry

My Cycles This Past Year
Shortest Cycle 35   Longest Cycle 45
Shortest Period 6   Longest Period 8

One thing to note is that she stopped observing her fluid after she found her Fluid Peak Day. It can be nice to take a break from doing observations, if you've gotten all the information you need from your chart! But we can take a look at her "Exercise" custom line and see that she met her exercise goals on Day 40, since that's checked off.

So we know that this cycle is at least 40 days long... but how do we know when this cycle ends? In an app, this is easy because it will split up your charts for you automatically, but paper charts are less flexible since they always show the same number of days. So, how do we know how long this cycle actually was? There can be different ways of keeping track of cycle lengths, but the easiest way is to add some sort of note on your chart when your new period begins. You could just write in the margin: "This cycle was 43 days long." You could also put a squiggly line through the last day of your cycle, or come up with your own unique way to mark the paper!

TROUBLESHOOTING CERVICAL FLUID

In this guide, we've learned a really simple way to classify cervical fluid observations. But there are other methods of observing and categorizing this fluid, and part of the reason different options exist is because girls' and women's bodies are different, and we have different preferences!

You've learned how to observe fluid by wiping and then looking at the results. But some methods of observing fluid don't even require you to look at the type of secretions: you just go based on the feeling. Or other methods will have you go into a lot more detail with your observations, to get more distinct categories.

So all this is to say: if for any reason you feel like this system of observing and charting fluid doesn't make immediate sense to you, that's alright. Maybe a different approach may work better for you.

It's also possible that you may feel like you NEVER have GRAY days, and you're always seeing YELLOW or TEAL. You could be wondering if something is wrong. Or maybe you feel like you almost always have GRAY observations and you never really feel like you're able to observe TEAL in order to find a Fluid Peak Day.

Even adults can have these issues! So try not to get discouraged if you feel like your body isn't showing you what you expect to see. What I'll offer here are some quick tips for observing fluid that might help if you find yourself feeling a little stuck:

Having a hard time remembering your fluid observations? Stack three bracelets as a visual reminder to check fluid when you use the bathroom. Move them around to keep track of fluid during the day. If one bracelet is closest to your hand, it means one category. If another bracelet is on top, it's a different category.

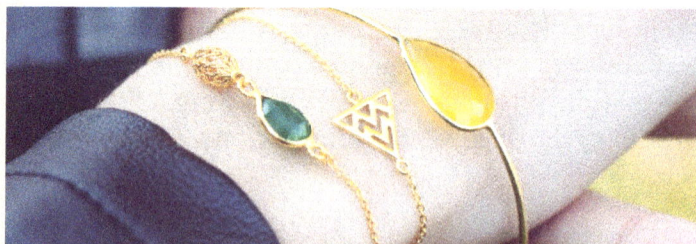

FLUID PRO TIPS

If you feel like you're **almost always GRAY**:
- Check your hydration levels! Our bodies need water to make fluid. It's possible that increasing water intake could lead to more obvious fluid signs.
- It can be easy to miss our fluid signs during the day because we're distracted with lots of other important things. So maybe pay attention to see if you have fluid after a bowel movement. That's a likely time when we might push out any fluid, even if just a little bit.
- If wiping isn't helpful, you might have better luck trying to notice different sensations as you walk around.
- Make sure you're not using scented toilet paper or wearing pantyliners which would actually dry up your external observations.

If you feel like you **never have a GRAY day:**
- That's actually okay! Remember that we can find Fluid Peak Day just by having YELLOW observations after TEAL. But if you're getting so much fluid that it's hard to find a Fluid Peak Day, this might not be a super helpful sign right now. OR you can modify your categories. Some girls and women have a lot of stretch all the time, so you might feel like you need to mark TEAL every day. But there could be a meaningful difference between stretchy fluid that is white or yellow, compared to stretchy fluid that's really clear and wet. So try marking the white/yellow stretchy stuff as YELLOW category to see if that makes Peak Day more obvious!

TROUBLESHOOTING TEMPS

If you are tracking temperatures, you may sometimes feel like you see a chart with no real temperature shift. Maybe there isn't a clear pattern of low temperatures and then high temperatures. It's possible that you could see this if you have an anovulatory bleed, because that would mean you haven't ovulated and therefore haven't produced any progesterone that would cause a shift.

OR, it's possible that you're not seeing shifts because high quality temperature data can admittedly be tricky to get. We already discussed that some forms of temping are just more accurate than others. So maybe it's a limitation of the device itself.

But temperatures can also be affected by a lot of things! If you're really hot one night while you're sleeping and then turn on the air conditioning the next night, that might affect your body temperature in the morning. Temperatures can also be less accurate if you aren't taking your temperature at the same time every morning, or if your sleep schedule changes a lot. So don't be too hard on yourself if your temperature line just looks crazy sometimes. That's okay.

What I'd like to offer here are a few tips for you to try **if you really want** to get better temperature accuracy.

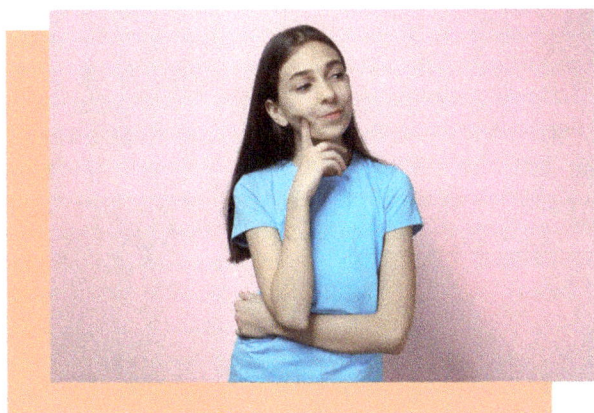

TEMPING PRO TIPS

If you are using a WEARABLE thermometer:
- check your thermometer placement, to ensure proper orientation of any sensors and that you are wearing the device in a suggested/approved location against your skin.
- make sure you are always using the same placement (e.g., not switching from left to right if it's watch, or switching fingers if it's a ring).
- ensure your device is properly charged
- if you suspect major errors, most companies will allow you to reach out for technical support and/or a data review.

If you are using an ORAL thermometer:
- check your thermometer placement, making sure that you're correctly putting the thermometer in the heat pocket under your tongue.
- make sure to breathe ONLY through your nose while the thermometer is reading
- take temps immediately upon waking (no sips of water first).
- consider sleeping with your thermometer under your pillow, so it stays a warm, consistent temperature over night.
- make sure you're getting at least three hours of uninterrupted sleep before taking your temperature.
- be as consistent as you can with your sleep schedule, so your waking time is about the same. This can be referred to as a **BASE TIME,** and if you're consistent enough about hitting your Base Time regularly, there are more tips on the next page that you can use for adjusting temperatures if you happen to miss your Base Time.

TROUBLESHOOTING TEMPS

If you are using an oral thermometer to track your BBT, you'll get the most accurate results if you have regular sleep and can hit a consistent **Base Time** for waking up. When you're on a regular schedule, this can be a pretty easy thing to do. But what about if you are on summer break? Or if you want to sleep in on the weekends? There's no need for you to stress out about getting the BEST temperature data possible. So you may just not want to worry about this at all! But if you want to get the best accuracy from your temperatures, you can accommodate variations in your schedule in one of the following ways:

1. if you want to sleep in a little, just set an alarm at your regular Base Time, take your temp, and then fall back asleep!
2. take your temperature whenever you wake up, but do some adjustments. If you do this, always note on your chart what time you woke up and what your original temperature reading was. You would chart the adjusted temperature value on the graph.

HOW DO ADJUSTMENTS WORK?

After hitting your lowest temperature of the night, your body raises its temperature by about a tenth of a degree Fahrenheit (one decimal point) every HALF HOUR as your body prepares to wake up. So for every half hour you sleep in, you subtract 0.1 to get back to what your temp **would have been** at your Base Time. For every half hour you get up early, you add 0.1 **to predict** what your temp would have been at your Base Time. Use the chart below to help:

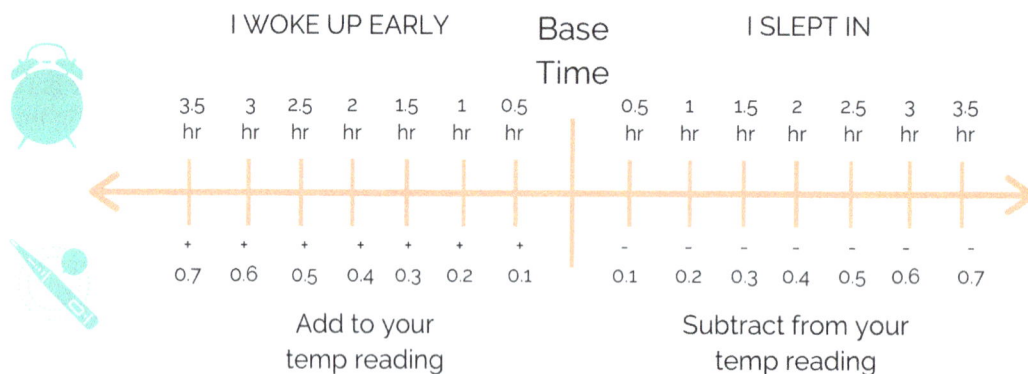

	I WOKE UP EARLY						Base Time		I SLEPT IN					
3.5 hr	3 hr	2.5 hr	2 hr	1.5 hr	1 hr	0.5 hr		0.5 hr	1 hr	1.5 hr	2 hr	2.5 hr	3 hr	3.5 hr
+ 0.7	+ 0.6	+ 0.5	+ 0.4	+ 0.3	+ 0.2	+ 0.1		- 0.1	- 0.2	- 0.3	- 0.4	- 0.5	- 0.6	- 0.7

Add to your temp reading | Subtract from your temp reading

Try some examples!

Monday
Base Time: 7:00 AM
Wake up time: 8:00 AM
Her thermometer read: 97.4°
She will chart: _____

Tuesday
Base Time: 7:00 AM
Wake up time: 8:30 AM
Her thermometer read: 97.8°
She will chart: _____

Help Maria fill out her chart!

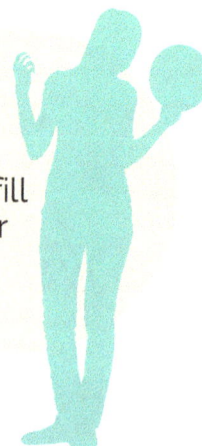

Wednesday
Base Time: 7:00 AM
Wake up time: 6:30 AM
Her thermometer read: 97.7°
She will chart: _____

Thursday
Base Time: 7:00 AM
Wake up time: 5:00 AM
Her thermometer read: 97.1°
She will chart: _____

Check your answers at the end of this book

TROUBLESHOOTING HORMONE HELP

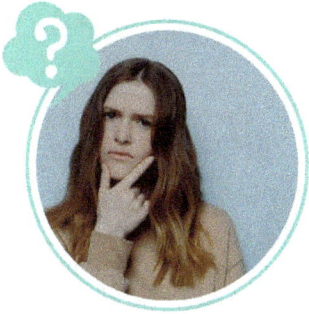

My doctor says that taking hormones will help me with some cycle symptoms I am having, and can even make my cycles more regular. They call this "birth control" but I don't really know what that is or what the different options are. Can that actually help me?

We already know that teen cycles and periods can be less regular than cycles and periods when you're grown up—the hormone ratios are just different, and the HPO axis is still figuring things out. So remember that there's no need to force your cycles to become more regular in the first few years. Your body is actually doing the really complicated work of learning how to put together a more regular cycle on its own, and that can just take some time.

But that doesn't mean that all of the symptoms and variations are easy to deal with all the time. It's possible for teens to have heavier bleeding, more bothersome cramps, acne, and mood swings—just to name a few issues. And it's not like middle school and high school are particularly easy times anyway: it seems really unfair if you have to navigate all of that at once!

So, it's definitely appropriate to speak with your doctor about helping you alleviate some of those other symptoms if it feels like they are interfering with your ability to function, or if they point towards any of the possible issues which are covered in the section on cycle health. You deserve to have your symptoms taken seriously.

Unfortunately, the most common way symptoms are managed is through synthetic hormones which actually override your body's HPO axis and replace your natural cycles with artificial ones. These sorts of drugs are ofter referred to as "birth control" because one of the main things they do is to prevent ovulation from happening, meaning pregnancy wouldn't be possible. There can certainly be moral concerns with this approach, but those get into deeper topics than this book can cover! So we will focus here specifically on reasons why girls may want to find a different medical treatment than birth control for their cycle health issues.

There are two main types of hormonal birth control, which can be delivered in different forms like pills, patches, or even long-lasting injections. The first type is progestin-only, which means that your body receives an artificial hormone which is kind of like progesterone. As long as you are taking the progestin, you won't have a bleed. If you take the hormone continuously, it's possible to skip having bleeds altogether.

The second type of hormonal birth control is often called "combined" hormones, which means it contains both estrogen and progestin. By supplying the body with a steady stream of these synthetic hormones, the drugs work to suppress ovulation and cause other changes which thin out cervical fluid and the uterine lining. When you stop taking the hormones, you will have a type of anovulatory bleed that we haven't talked about before because it only happens artificially with these drugs: a synthetic hormone withdrawal bleed. It's not a real period because ovulation hasn't happened, but it mimics a natural period because it is caused by a drop in estrogen and progesterone.

TROUBLESHOOTING HORMONE HELP

Another type of birth control option you should be aware of is something called an intrauterine device, or IUD for short. These devices are surgically implanted into the uterus and come in two types as well: hormonal, or non-hormonal.

The hormonal IUD is basically just a different delivery system for the progestin-only option we discussed above. The non-hormonal IUD is a copper coil, which does not override your natural cycles and does not prevent ovulation. Instead, it makes the uterus a hostile environment for pregnancy by initiating an inflammatory response, thinning the uterine lining, and changing cervical fluid.

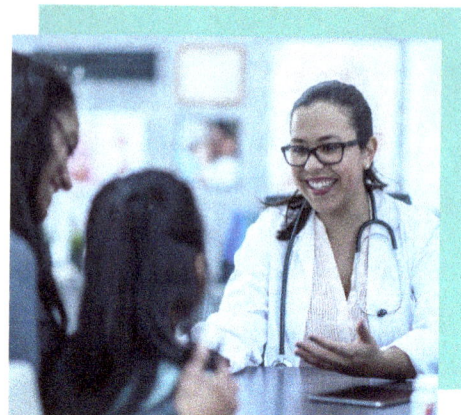

If you are experiencing difficult cycle symptoms, it is unlikely that your doctor would recommend a copper IUD, because it does not contain any hormones. But if you are having certain symptoms associated with your cycles, a doctor might suggest you utilize some of the synthetic hormone options. In cases where hormone imbalances were the major thing contributing to symptoms, it's possible that these synthetic options may alleviate or improve the issues you were having. **But hopefully at this point, you have a good understanding of why ovulation is healthy for girls' bodies and why it might be a good idea to help your HPO axis mature on its own rather than overriding it and effectively shutting it down.** This should definitely be a part of the conversation you have with your doctor, because finding the right treatment or management plan for your situation should include honest conversations about the benefits and risks involved. And taking synthetic hormones can come with a big list of risks like blood clots, increased risk for certain cancers, nausea, headaches, or depression. So don't be afraid to ask those questions!

But you should also know that there are ways to supplement hormones more gently, by working in a cooperative way with your cycle (instead of overriding it). Another hormonal option which is less common for doctors to suggest is called **bioidentical hormone therapy.** These hormones are also synthetic because they are produced in a lab, but they have a chemical structure which matches your natural hormones so it's possible for them to be gentler and in some cases, to carry fewer risks. Additionally, bioidentical hormones can be used in a cooperative way with your cycles. So, because you have learned how to chart your cycles to look for ovulation, you'd likely be able to take bioidentical hormones in a way that can keep your natural cycles intact, for example: by waiting until ovulation has been confirmed to take progesterone supplements, when it is naturally appropriate for that hormone to be in your body.

You can refer to the list of resources from the health section to find doctors that are more likely to take this sort of approach, sometimes called **Restorative Reproductive Medicine,** because the goal of this style of treatment is to support the natural menstrual cycle rather than overriding it. However, please know that it can be very difficult to get this level of support. Telehealth options have certainly made it easier! But if you are suffering with severe symptoms and the best option you have available to you are the more potent synthetic hormones, there is nothing morally wrong about using them for relief. Just remember that if there is an underlying condition causing cycle issues: birth control will not solve it, comes with medical risks, and you will still probably have to tackle the difficult task of digging deeper at some point to get real resolution.

CONCLUSION

Dear girls,

Congratulations!! You have learned SO much about your body and about how to observe its unique cycle signs—but this is just the beginning! Coming to know and appreciate your body is something that everyone goes through during puberty, but it's also a lifelong process we continue to go through as we age and our bodies keep changing. Eventually, your body will go through **menopause (MEH-nuh-paaz)** and stop cycling, which will be another opportunity to keep learning!

It is a great achievement to be able to appreciate the work your body does, throughout all the ups and downs of life. You should be proud that you have worked so hard to become educated and equipped with knowledge about your menstrual cycle. Just remember: it takes a long time to learn to "read" the signs that your body is giving you. So be patient with yourself as you begin to chart.

If you ever have questions, I hope you feel empowered to ask for help from a trusted adult, or from a friend. Likewise, remember that you have lots of knowledge that can help your friends if *they* have questions. I encourage all of you to work to build a Culture of Care for one another — so that every girl can learn to understand, respect, and appreciate her unique body!

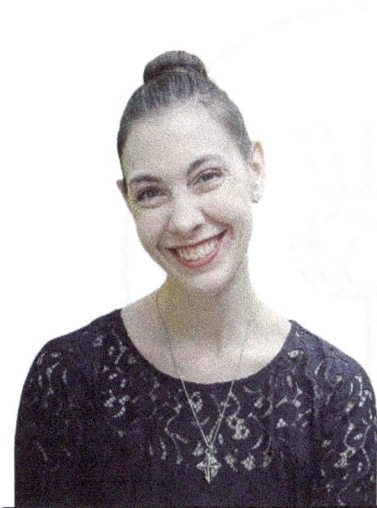

Christina Valenzuela
owner- Pearl & Thistle

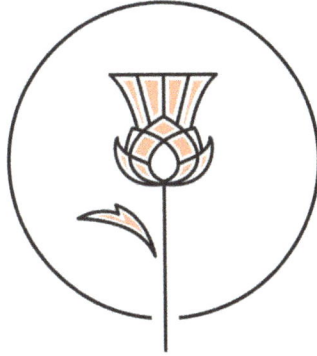

CHARTS

*PDF downloads of these charts are available
in the Pearl & Thistle shop online:*
pearlandthistle.com

THIS CHART BELONGS TO: _____

CYCLE START DATE: _____   MY CUSTOM FIELDS: _____

CYCLE END DATE: _____   _____

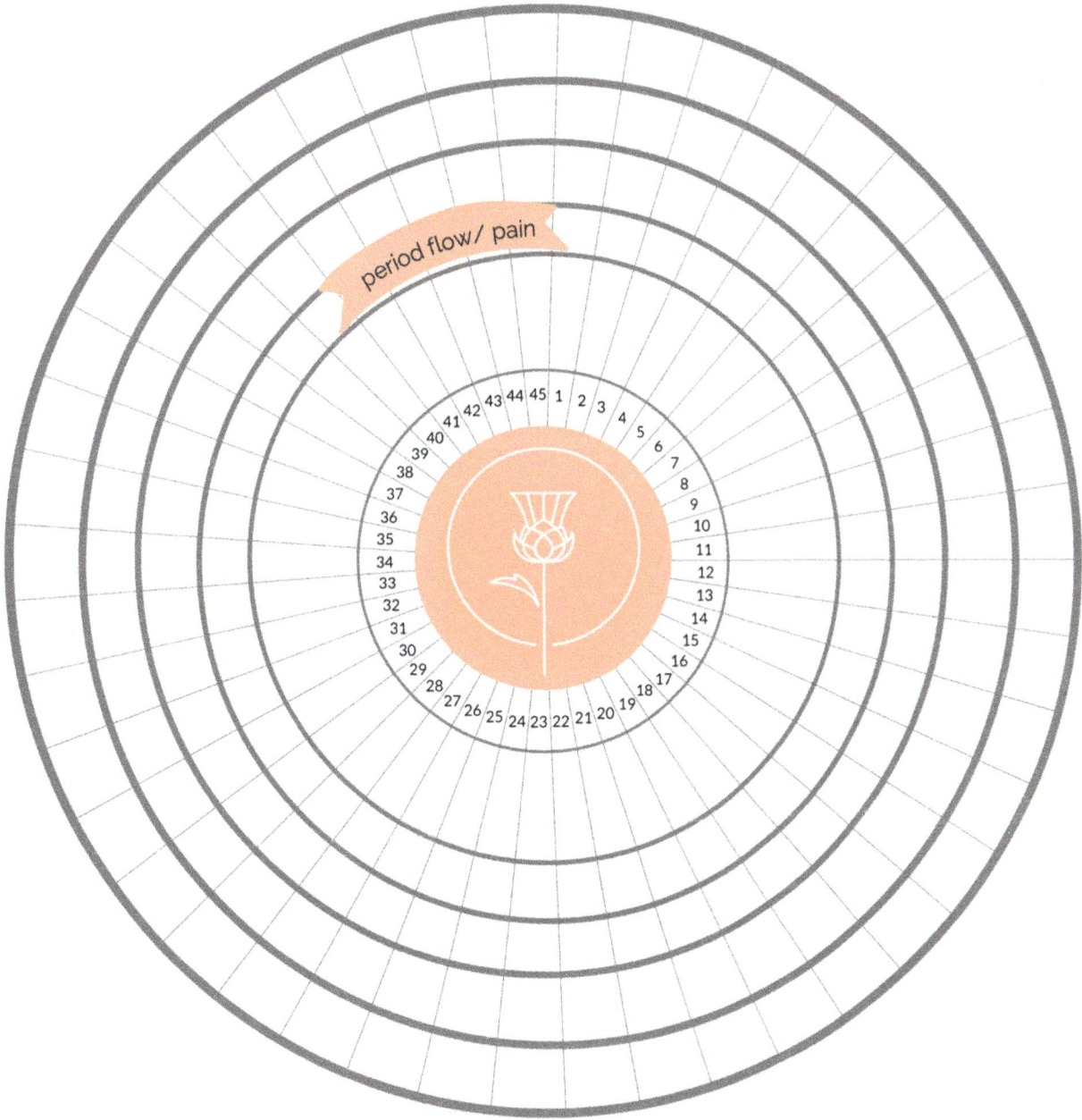

period flow/ pain

41 42 43 44 45 1 2 3 4 5 6 7 8 9 10 11 12 13 14 15 16 17 18 19 20 21 22 23 24 25 26 27 28 29 30 31 32 33 34 35 36 37 38 39 40

Color Codes:
Red = flow of blood
Red dots= spotting
Gray = dry, no fluid
Yellow = moist/sticky, pasty, creamy, slightly stretchy fluid
Teal = slippery/wet, clear, stretchy, slippery, watery fluid

Period:
L= light flow
M= moderate flow
H= heavy flow
Pain:
0= no pain
1= little bit uncomfortable
2= moderate discomfort
3= pain interferes with my day

Mood:
+ = happy
☆ = neutral
= angry
-- = sad
@ = stressed

add your own!

Chart 1

Date																																													
---	1	2	3	4	5	6	7	8	9	10	11	12	13	14	15	16	17	18	19	20	21	22	23	24	25	26	27	28	29	30	31	32	33	34	35	36	37	38	39	40	41	42	43	44	45
Day of Cycle																																													
Period & Fluid																																													
Fluid Notations																																													
Period Pain?																																													
My Mood																																													

Chart 2

Date																																													
---	1	2	3	4	5	6	7	8	9	10	11	12	13	14	15	16	17	18	19	20	21	22	23	24	25	26	27	28	29	30	31	32	33	34	35	36	37	38	39	40	41	42	43	44	45
Day of Cycle																																													
Period & Fluid																																													
Fluid Notations																																													
Period Pain?																																													
My Mood																																													

Chart 3

Date																																													
---	1	2	3	4	5	6	7	8	9	10	11	12	13	14	15	16	17	18	19	20	21	22	23	24	25	26	27	28	29	30	31	32	33	34	35	36	37	38	39	40	41	42	43	44	45
Day of Cycle																																													
Period & Fluid																																													
Fluid Notations																																													
Period Pain?																																													
My Mood																																													

KEY

Fluid Notations

L= Light Flow   M= Moderate Flow   H = Heavy Flow

Period & Fluid

Red = flow of blood   Dots = spotting   Gray = dry, no fluid

Yellow = moist/sticky, pasty, creamy, slightly stretchy fluid

Teal = slippery/wet, clear, stretchy, slippery, watery fluid

Period Pain

0 = no pain

1 = a little uncomfortable

2 = medium amount of discomfort

3 = pain interferes with my day

Mood

+ = Happy

☆ = Neutral

-- = Sad

@ = Stressed

= Angry

pearlandthistle.com

Date																																												
Day of Cycle	1	2	3	4	5	6	7	8	9	10	11	12	13	14	15	16	17	18	19	20	21	22	23	24	25	26	27	28	29	30	31	32	33	34	35	36	37	38	39	40	41	42	43	44	45

Year _____

Temperature grid rows: 98, 9, 8, 7, 6, 5, 4, 3, 2, 1, 97, 9, 8, 7, 6, 5, 4, 3, 2, 1, 96

Cycle # _____

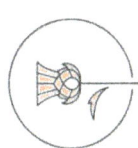

My Cycles This Past Year

Shortest Cycle _____   Longest Cycle _____

Shortest Period _____   Longest Period _____

A COUPLE OF EXTRA RESOURCES...

Would you like to read more about the menstrual cycle? Check out:
What's Going on in My Body? : All about the Female Cycle, Periods and Fertility by Elisabeth Raith-Paula, M.D.

If you are looking for a free app alternative to Ready Your Body, you can check out the FEMM app. Visit **femmhealth.org** for more info. The fluid categories do not line up perfectly with what we have learned here— both "pasty" and "moist" categories would be the equivalent of our "YELLOW."

SELECTED BIBLIOGRAPHY:

- American College of Obstetricians and Gynecologists, Committee Opinion Number 651, "Menstruation in Girls and Adolescents: Using the Menstrual Cycle as a Vital Sign," acog.org, Dec 2015.
- Billings LIFE, "Normal Types of Bleeding," billings.life/en/, 2023.
- Briden, Lara. *Period Repair Manual.* Green Peak Publishing, 2018.
- Centers for Disease Control and Prevention, "Are You Getting Enough Sleep?" cdc.gov, Apr 2021.
- Hendrickson-Jack, Lisa. *The Fifth Vital Sign.* Fertility Friday Publishing, 2019.
- Knight, Jane. *The Complete Guide to Fertility Awareness.* Oxon: Routledge, 2017.
- Metten, Shelley and Alan Estridge. *I'm a Girl: Hormones!* Anatomy for Kids, 2018.
- McCracken, Katherine. "Menstruation in Adolescents: The Importance of Using Menses as a Vital Sign," www.nationwidechildrens.org, Jul 2019.
- Natterson, Cara. *The Care & Keeping of You 2: The Body Book for Older Girls.* American Girl Publishing, 2018.
- Raith-Paula, Elisabeth. *What's Going On In My Body?.* Hungary: Gerhard Paula MFM PrintMedia, 2018.
- Schaefer, Valorie Lee. *The Care & Keeping of You 1: The Body Book for Younger Girls.* American Girl Publishing, 2018.
- Shannon, Marilyn M. *Fertility, Cycles & Nutrition.* Cincinnati: Couple to Couple League International, Inc., 2009.
- Weschler, Toni. *Cycle Savvy.* New York: HarperCollins Publishers, 2006.

Fluid charting answers:

Tuesday:	Wednesday:	Thursday:
Yellow	Teal	Yellow
Yellow	Teal	Yellow
Teal	Teal	Gray
Teal	Teal	Gray
TEAL	TEAL	YELLOW

Temp adjustment worksheet answers:

Monday: 97.2°
Tuesday: 97.5°
Wednesday: 97.8°
Thursday: 97.5°